Pretty
Takes
Practice

Pretty
Takes
Practice

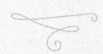

CHARLA MULLER

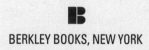

BERKLEY BOOKS, NEW YORK

THE BERKLEY PUBLISHING GROUP
Published by the Penguin Group
Penguin Group (USA) LLC
375 Hudson Street, New York, New York 10014

USA • Canada • UK • Ireland • Australia • New Zealand • India • South Africa • China

penguin.com

A Penguin Random House Company

This book is an original publication of The Berkley Publishing Group.

Library of Congress Cataloging-in-Publication Data

Muller, Charla.
Pretty takes practice : a southern woman's search for the real meaning of beauty / Charla Muller.
p. cm.
ISBN 978-0-425-26619-9 (paperback)
1. Body image.   2. Beauty, Personal—Psychological aspects.
3. Beauty, Personal—Humor.   I. Title.
BF697.5.B63M85   2014
646.7001'9—dc23   2014010563

PUBLISHING HISTORY
Berkley trade paperback edition / August 2014

PRINTED IN THE UNITED STATES OF AMERICA

10 9 8 7 6 5 4 3 2 1

Cover photos: (front) © 1858. All rights reserved. Originally published in *Glamour*.
Reprinted by permission. (back) Powder box and roses © Andrii Muzyka / Shutterstock.
Cover design by Danielle Abbiate.
Interior text design by Laura K. Corless.

To my mother

ACKNOWLEDGMENTS

I'd like to thank Brandi Bowles, my agent, for taking a chance on an author's sophomore book.

And to Andie Avila, who again offered her gentle hand to firmly guide me.

To my writing buddies, Judy Goldman and Betsy Thorpe, who helped me wrestle this idea into a book proposal. Writing groups are often just therapy sessions in disguise and this was no different. Thank you for your encouragement and tough love.

To my dearest friends, many of whom are featured here. We all have tales of pretty, and I am grateful for such beautiful, talented and authentic friends. Special thanks to my sister-in-law, Kathleen, who always offered a hand, an ear and a shoulder.

To Brad and my two terrific kids—your willingness to indulge me defies belief.

And to my mother, who has led a life worthy of example when it comes to pretty, both inside and out.

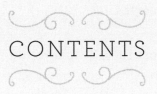

CONTENTS

INTRODUCTION

The Importance of Being Pretty

I live in a city that is bright and glossy, with modern skyscrapers that glitter and twinkle, seeming to invite you to join in the polished success of our fair metropolis. Pretty and freshly renovated houses sit perched on wide, tree-lined streets and beckon you to daydream about their finely appointed interiors. Gorgeously landscaped yards boast perfectly placed azaleas, magnolia trees and crepe myrtles and bid you to come lounge in their shade. Shiny new SUVs, smart cars, MINI Coopers and luxury sedans buzz around town to appointments, meetings, carpools, bridge games and tennis matches. And in those skyscrapers, houses, yards and cars are very attractive, well-groomed and nicely dressed women who took the time and the energy to get pretty.

Pretty girls are everywhere in my town of Charlotte, North Carolina. Case in point—my girlfriend's best pal visits annually from New York City: the world's epicenter of all things sleek, chic and au courant. And what does she say when it's time to leave the Queen City of Charlotte? "I can't wait to get out of here—

everyone is so damned attractive, it totally bums me out." Don't I know it, friend. This town is ruining the curve on pretty. When one is a really-very-average-middle-aged mom living in a city where pretty reigns and grooming is high art, looking put together and feeling pulled together can be more challenging than pumping and freezing six months' worth of breast milk in a feeble attempt to bulletproof the immune system of my babies (who are now sneaking full-leaded soda from vending machines).

Many of us live in a Pretty City somewhere, and the pressure to look great more days than not can be crippling. And until the day I published a book, appeared on national television and subjected myself to input from the collective universe, I really was okay with looking fairly decent about every third day. Hitting a self-imposed beauty bar 30 percent of the time felt pretty good. And I did have a beauty bar, mind you. I am a southerner born and bred, and schooled in appropriate grooming (including facial hair management), good manners (lots of "yes ma'ams" and "no sirs") and sound fashion habits (no wind suits on airplanes). Even as a full-time working mom I was happy to exceed that bar for big client presentations and power lunches. And the rest of the time, I could and would slack off the grooming gas a little and coast. I still presented fairly well and had some basic requisites: No baseball caps—EVER! Clean face and fresh makeup every morning. Skirts and Dansko clogs are not meant to be worn at the same time, I don't care if you are a librarian at a Montessori school (which I'm not).

I aspired to a certain level of pretty and knew enough fundamentals to head in the right direction; I was just admittedly and selectively inconsistent. But appearing on national television forever changed my thinking about appearances as well as my apparent delusion that one out of every three days of aspiring to present well was good enough.

You see, several years ago I wrote a memoir about the year of daily intimacy I gave my husband, Brad, for his fortieth birthday. This randy little tale raised a few eyebrows (especially in my neck of the woods) and caught the attention of the media. *People* magazine, the *Today* show, CNN and *The View* came calling, which is every publisher's dream and certainly a first-time author's dream, too. And while I was eager to share my message and promote my book, I quickly learned what everyone really wanted to know. The very first question on everybody's lips before appearing anywhere was not what this newly minted author was going to *say*, but rather: what would a wife who offered her husband daily intimacy for an entire year *look* like? I was forced to confront the reality that people might not care what I had to say if they couldn't get past how I looked. And so I tried mightily to present with as much confidence as I could muster with a very stocky frame and some serious postbaby weight tucked behind a well-tailored skirt, a sassy scarf and flats (no Dansko clogs).

Don't get me wrong, I was flattered that people had taken an interest in my experience and what I had to share about marriage. I was confident that my husband appreciated the gift (even if I was a few pounds heavier than when we were first married), and hoped my message—more intimacy within marriage is transformative—would provoke meaningful conversations. And of course, sitting next to Whoopi Goldberg in the makeup chair and kibitzing with Elisabeth Hasselbeck and Barbara Walters before sailing out to sit with all the girls on *The View* is pretty amazing. So sure, all of the publicity was fabulous—*in the abstract . . . and then when it was over.* But when it's actually happening to you (yes, you!) at that very moment, in real time, it's the kind of experience that can reduce you to the most fundamental of female fears, which is, of course, *holy mother of Frédéric Fekkai, how do I look?*

Like it or not, how I looked determined my credibility to the viewing and reading audience. It determined my likability, and ultimately, my salability. While others who randomly tripped over me in an article or on national television could—if they so wanted—scrutinize me, my message and looks, I spent the better part of a year turning away from the magazine articles, the national television segments and the newspaper photos. I knew what I looked like and I didn't need to study, analyze or obsess over it. After all, I had places to go and people to see, like Oprah.

I was invited to appear on *The Oprah Winfrey Show*, which was an honor—even if you're being Skyped in from your living room sitting on your sofa, under the light of shadeless table lamps, sweating off a full face of makeup for fifty-five minutes (which feels like fifty-five dog years, by the way) until your segment tapes in minute fifty-six. I repeat, this was a true honor and I would do it again in a heartbeat. Though I'd do it differently because let me tell you, watching yourself LIVE on the giant screen behind Oprah's rather large but well-coiffed head is like watching your own car accident . . . or your own birth. It's simply something you shouldn't witness.

I stared at myself and wondered: *Is that me? Is that what my hair looks like, really? Does it always swing in such an awkward way when I move my head? Did I actually think that black knit sweater would hide the extra sixty pounds I've been lugging around? I think I bought that sweater five years ago at Stein Mart—why would I wear a five-year-old knit sweater from Steinie on the freakin'* Oprah Winfrey Show? *Why is my lipstick so dark? I look like Elvira. Can I sue Oprah and demand she not run this segment? Can Brad divorce me on the grounds of public humiliation on national television?*

Well, you get the idea.

On that giant screen behind Oprah's head I looked like a giant, bloated mess—a tough thing to witness in real time when I'm trying to appear poised and articulate in front of O and the rest of the free world. Not to mention incredibly distracting. And lest you think I'm exaggerating about or overreacting to my appearance, let me tell you that I had plenty of unadoring fans reassure me that I wasn't.

Let me also add that I'm all about large doses of reality that force some much-needed personal introspection—after all, I was the one to admit that my marriage had lost a little of its bedroom ooomph. But doing it LIVE in front of ten million people kinda stinks. It turned out that my 30 percent wasn't cutting it, despite my efforts to exceed my beauty bar during a moment when it really mattered. Sure, I was busy offering my husband every man's dream gift, working on marketing campaigns, meeting the school bus and throwing some awesome dinner parties in the year leading up to this event of sorts. But reflecting back, I realize that I had allowed those things to consume me and didn't concern myself with much else. Clearly I had been neglecting myself and in the process drifting off course into a sea of denial. In other words: while I was presenting well in the bedroom (behind closed doors and in the dark), I clearly wasn't working hard enough to present to the world. Denial, much?

Denial is built into my DNA. I get it from my father's side. And I must add, they were a pretty contented bunch. They all lived in a happy little place where everyone stays happily married, no one has children out of wedlock, no one drinks too much, no one talks behind your back and that tree in the backyard is always growing money.

Kind of like Cosette's sweet little song from *Les Misérables*: "Nobody shouts or talks too loud, not in my castle on a cloud." Amen, sister. In my castle on a cloud, no one notices the fact that they've never seen me in a pair of denim jeans or that the statute of limitations on baby weight expired when my son started kindergarten or that my eyebrows often resemble mating caterpillars.

But I couldn't go on in denial once I was confronted (finally) with the image of the "Real Charla." The truth is that what doesn't kill you, or drive you to vow to never leave your house during daylight hours, might possibly give you a little perspective. In a very real way, it was like surviving a tornado—I emerged stunned, disoriented, and changed (in ways, mind you, that I'm convinced I've not yet pinpointed completely) . . . and with a new hairstyle. After surviving the storm of criticism, scrutiny and even some late-night commentary, I found out that I could handle a bit more of the real world than perhaps I cared to handle. Combine that insight with a slow dance into middle age, and what you've got is not always a life-affirming combination but rather a strange, uncomfortable intersection of self-awareness and resignation. It was an Accidental Beauty Intervention of sorts. What I saw changed me. First, I cried. I admit it. (Call me a thin-skinned, self-absorbed preteen, but you try watching yourself on live television in front of ten million people at age forty-three. Then you call me, okay? We'll chat.) Then I bucked up and got to it. I joined a weight-loss program, started eating better and exercising, and gradually shed pounds. About the equivalent of a second grader. That felt good, I have to say. I went shopping and upgraded my closet with current (and much smaller) frocks. And I rediscovered some of the beauty basics that I had either forgotten or repressed.

All told, confronting my personal image was a good thing. Because for a long time, despite the fact that I avoided the scale, I knew the scale didn't lie. And neither did the sales associates in the store who brought impossibly sized clothes to my dressing room while I swallowed my pride (and a few Xanax). And neither did my mother when she would sigh out a comment like a long exhale from a cigarette she no longer smokes. "Oh, sweetie, you have such a beautiful face . . ." *Whatever.*

Whether we care to admit it or not, our ideas of beauty and appearance help us make order of our lives. Which is why villains are ugly, heroines are beautiful, funny sidekicks are round and *never* get the girl (or guy) and mean, spinster schoolteachers are tall, spindly and old. We can visually organize our world if our assumptions about beauty and appearance are universally true. We know where we stand—in our family and in our school and in our garden club. This is why the Ugly Duckling has collective meaning for us all. This is also why I care. (And why deep down you do, too.)

As it turns out, first impressions count, size matters, grace and manners are noticed, playing to your strengths makes a difference and your mother's little tips on getting pretty are likely spot-on. The truth is, it's easy to not concern yourself with all this stuff, but it is important. It doesn't matter more than some things, like health, God, positive relationships with family and friends, finding a purpose, having a roof over your head and food on the table and a world without twerking, but it can matter enough to inform and impact those things, for better and for worse.

Post *Oprah* (yes, there is life after *O*), I spent two years working hard—to spiff up the inside and the out. It would be easy to sum up my experience as the oh-so-expected, maudlin exercise of some vain, washed-up southern suburban working mom. But I found it forced more out of me than a regular meet-up with my dermatologist or a clothing date with my overstuffed closet.

Seeing yourself for the first time not as you think others see you but as they actually do see you, forced me, at the age of forty-three, to grow up.

It forced me to acknowledge a deeper truth about the power of appearance, beyond the frivolous and sometimes stereotypical mantle that southern women wear. It forced me to reconcile what I thought I looked like with what I really did look like. It forced me to raise my beauty bar—not because others bullied me to raise it but rather because I knew I *could* and I wanted to know what that would feel and look like. It forced me to sift through all my emotional baggage about beauty, appearance and my mother (a source of all good baggage) and decide what I was going to own and what I was going to pack away for good. It forced me to take a different kind of stand on getting pretty. And it made me realize that while getting pretty is not the pursuit of perfection, it is the pursuit of an appreciation for and an understanding of the different layers and nuances that make us all inimitably pretty. And most important, it forced me to realize that pretty, at least my definition of it, takes practice. Inside and out.

This book is not a how-to guide on how to achieve pretty. Nor is it a chronological account of my own "transformation." After all, I'm still figuring it out—you know, good personal growth and transformation days, bad personal growth and transformation days and all that. My story is messy, misguided and, at times, tragically comic. Instead what follows are reflections on some experiences over the course of many years that led me to determine my own list of rules for what it takes to feel pretty, stay pretty and possibly die pretty (but I'm not that far in the story yet).

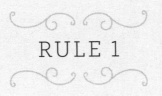

RULE 1

*Looking Good Takes Time,
So Find Some*

I have a vivid memory of my mother and a spectacular pair of sunglasses. They had black and white stripes and giant black lenses, and instead of an earpiece, there was a delicate chain that draped behind each ear, weighted down by a black-and-white disc that served double duty as . . . are you ready? An earring! Can you stand it? Eyewear as fashion accessory—eat your heart out, Foster Grant!

It was 1973, and my mother looked fabulous. I was only six at the time, but I knew it. Or rather, I felt it, as if by instinct—a primal knowledge of sorts. My heart swelled with happiness as I snuggled up against her legs while she poked through the clothing racks at Connie's Tru-Fit Fashions on Merrimon Avenue in the heart of Asheville, North Carolina.

My mother was pretty.

I watched my mother thoughtfully sorting through those racks of polyester, cotton and wool-blend items—pulling out clothes, giving them an appraising look, draping possibilities over her left arm. I felt a sense of pride over a discovery that I couldn't quite articulate but certainly recognized in the way salespeople approached her. It was the same way policemen told her to drive safely as they let her off with just a warning and how my classmates reacted to her when she brought in cupcakes and choreographed class parties. I imagined myself my mother's age, shopping for fabulous outfits. Like her, my charm bracelet would jingle jangle as I juggled hangers of clothes and flitted around nicely appointed stores and boutiques. In our small mountain town in the seventies, keeping up appearances had become high art.

What I didn't know then but would eventually discover was that there was much to learn when it came to the art of getting and feeling pretty. Fast-forward to when I was in junior high school and my mother and I were in a small dressing room at a different department store. This time, I was the one trying on clothes and schlepping down the hall outside the dressing room for a maternal once-over. My mother quietly studied me in the three-way mirror, her eyes scanning me from top to bottom and back up again.

"You're high-hipped," my mother finally announced. It was a declarative statement, as if she were teaching a master class on the art of well-tailored clothing (instead of just me, standing in a dressing room hallway, wearing a pair of pants that pooled around my feet). "You will always need to get your skirts hemmed *correctly* and your pants tapered *just so.*" She turned to confirm with the saleslady if the store alterationist was on hand.

I had little understanding of and appreciation for this little nugget, nor any of the others she cast my way during my awkward adolescence. At the time, I just wanted to BE pretty and not have to fuss with any of the more cumbersome and time-consuming details. I didn't want to admit that a lot of this pretty business took effort, especially when my first pretty memories were of my mother hosting glittery cocktail parties in an equally glittering one-piece pantsuit; or my mother lying by the pool in a bikini with a matching scarf tied around her hair and a cigarette in her hand; or my father's face when it lit up with pride and adoration as he slipped his arm around her narrow waist and escorted her to a party at the club. My mother made it all look so easy.

It wasn't until I was an adult that, in a moment of profound retribution, I realized my mother was right about my hips, never mind all the other things. For instance, skirts often sat lopsided on me. A pair of pants (or "slacks," as my mother liked to call them) didn't "fall" quite right. Blazers bunched on my short-waisted frame. I worked to pluck my mother's tutorials from the backseat of my memories in an effort to self-correct. That's when I ended up meeting Marine Sergeant Marie.

Marine Sergeant Marie was recommended by my friend Karen. The contrast between Karen and me is stark. She is nearly six feet tall and model thin. I am nearly five foot three and not. But the one thing we DID have in common is that neither of us dressed "off the rack" with great success, creating a pressing need for a high-quality dependable alterationist.

"I'd be happy to pass along my alteration lady's contact information," Karen shared one afternoon after a girls' birthday luncheon. We were chatting about spring wardrobe essentials and lamenting about the need for alterations. "But be warned. She's kind of brutal and to the point. And she's not cheap."

I took down Marine Sergeant Marie's number, confirmed her address and loaded my big honkin' SUV with clothes for my lunchtime appointment. She opened the door, and efficiently showed me into the bedroom–turned–sewing studio. She hung my clothes on a rack in her narrow hallway and sent me to her guest bathroom to get changed. Marie was a trim, attractive, single sixty-something with white-blond hair cut short.

She spent the first ten minutes circling, assessing and clucking under her breath. It was as if I were in a time machine that took me back three decades and I was standing there with my mother. "Well, let me get a look at you," she said, finally stopping to stand behind me, looking at me in the mirror that ran the length of her workroom. That's right, a mirror as big as an entire wall. While she stood behind me and we studied my reflection together, my palms started to sweat. Maybe the Asian ladies who spoke nada English and hemmed everything too short weren't all that bad, I thought to myself. They never made me pit out.

"Head up! Shoulders back," she barked. "You're too short to slouch. Don't stand with your knees locked, for God's sake, give your body some form."

She was right, but it was as if she was channeling my mother, my grandmother AND Joan Crawford (but without the hangers).

"What do you see when you look in the mirror?" she asked.

That was a trick question, I was sure of it. Marine Sergeant

Marie was going to make me do a hundred burpees if I didn't get this right. But I was stumped, so I just stood there.

"Quit acting like you want to disappear. Stand up and own the room." What she didn't know was that I did want to disappear. It was sensory overload—the mirror that allowed for no escape. Her sharp orders and firm instructions. For Pete's sake, I just needed her to fix my clothes; I had no idea she would try to fix me. But she kept tugging, pulling, pinning and lecturing. And then she started tucking and hemming and nipping, and sure enough, ill-fitting clothes started to take shape. Along the way, I picked up a tip or two, adding to and rounding out my mother's early instruction. Apparently lifelong learning doesn't apply just to one's career. It applies to getting pretty, too.

Years before Karen shared Marine Sergeant Marie with me and her need for fashion help, I was slightly stunned to discover that even the genetically blessed have to *work* to maintain the pretty—it's not just a happy accident. My college roommate was Malibu Barbie by way of Long Island. Really, she was (and still is) that pretty—pale blue eyes, a gorgeous smile with white teeth as straight as a picket fence and blond hair so thick that a ponytail holder would barely wrap around it twice. The only way to improve on her tanned and beachy good looks would be a tanned, beachy and equally handsome boyfriend. Enter stage left, handsome-surfer-boy-actor, whom she later married. (Yes, their children are genetically gifted, too.) Our senior year in college we were sitting around the sorority house, sporting baggy gym shorts and oversize fraternity T-shirts that boasted our popularity (or not), waxing poetic about some lame beauty conundrum—because, really, what beauty conundrum can you possibly have when you're twenty-one, blonde, tan and gorgeous (her, not me)?

That's when my roommate, Susan, the beach goddess, announced, "Just remember, girls, after the age of eighteen, there's no such thing as a natural blonde."

I think time skipped a second. I mean, I knew what girls like ME had to contend with (Jolene cream bleach and no hip-hugger jeans, for example), but I can honestly say that it never had occurred to me that even the preternaturally pretty had to manage their pretty, too. Ever since then, I've been a bit more sympathetic to my gorgeous sisters, trying to remember that we all have our various pretty priorities. Highlighting tresses to recall the sun-kissed color of youth. Monthly facial appointments in a quest for peachy-soft skin. Can't-miss dates with a personal trainer for a well-rounded booty. We're all force-ranking our beauty priorities based on our pretty preferences and the age-old truism that there is not enough time in the day to do it all.

From the day we are born ("the baby looks like me!") until the day we die ("she looks so peaceful"), people are judged on their looks. You do it. I do it. We all do it. We notice things, we assess things and we draw conclusions from these things. Or as my grandmother might say, "She didn't spend much time getting pretty today, now, did she?" And often these things do take time, don't they?

This is why one day my friend Kim arrived late to our bridge lesson. She took her seat at the square card table in the corner room of the Bridge Center, a former rec center–turned–card-playing safe house for bridge newbies and veterans. About a dozen women from thirty-five to fifty-five were crowded in the room, intent on learning nuances like no-trump interference bidding.

"Sorry," she whispered as she picked up her cards. "I was getting dressed for my annual. It's later today." My two girl-friends and I nodded and murmured conspiratorially in agree-ment and then counted our high-card points. Kim got a late pass that day—after all, annual physicals are like first dates and job interviews. They require time and focus.

There's no question I treat my annual exam like Date Night with my husband—the only difference is that one includes a speculum. First, I shower and shave—I shave everything that might need shaving, and even those parts that don't, just for good measure. Remember that preschool ditty "Head, Shoulders, Knees and Toes, Knees and Toes"? That's me with a razor. I'm shaving, looking, peering for anything weird or gross—as if my doctor has some delicate sensibility and might be grossed out by that mole, or that hair sprouting out of a mole. I loofah. I wash my hair, I condition my hair. Then I give my hair a nice long blowout. I put lotion all over, taking special care with my elbows and knees. My doc (who's a woman, mind you) doesn't care about my underwear. In fact, she doesn't even see my underwear—I'll be in a chilly little paper gown that's been wrinkled and shred-ded in my attempt to put it on the right way (it opens in the back, doesn't it?).

Charla Muller

But my underwear should be clean and fairly new anyway, right? God forbid I end up in a terrible accident on the way to the doctor and some ER nurse whom I know from my child's school might have to cut off my clothes and would instantly judge my skuzzy granny panties and not only deny me care, but also my rightful place on the PTA board next year. However, if I wear my new, personally-fitted-by-a-licensed-bra-fitter Wacoal Bra in a subtle neutral, the nurse would not only decide NOT to cut that high-quality, hand-washed undergarment from my body while I lay in the ER in need of a right lung, but also decide unequivocally that I should be PTA president (which I don't want to be, by the way). Really.

Lastly, I do my full makeup routine and put on nice jewelry for my doctor. I don't do perfume, though. Don't want her to think I'm trying too hard.

I want to look nice for my doctor. Healthy. Glowing. Youthful. Un-sick. I want her to see that I'm taking good care of myself, despite my overconsumption of wine on Saturday night and my overconsumption of the Red Velvet Pancake special at the IHOP on Sunday morning. I want her to compliment my cholesterol levels and approve of my exercise regimen and be blown away by my fabulous blood pressure. All told, I want my doctor to *approve*. As if her acknowledgment of my efforts to look good will negate all the things I'm NOT doing right.

The irony, of course, is that the time I took to get ready to see my doctor exceeded the time spent with my doctor by twofold. But that is irrelevant, because my goal is to look as great as this forty-something, full-time working mom of two on a part-time beauty budget can look these days. And let me tell you, at my last annual, I looked great! In fact, I hadn't looked that nice during daytime hours in such a long time that I called up Brad.

"Hey! I'm having my annual today and I look surprisingly great. Wanna meet me for lunch? I would hate for all this work to go to waste on Dr. Cole." So we did. Carpe diem, I say.

It's important for my primary-care doctor to approve of me, because five years earlier my ob-gyn unceremoniously dumped me. It took her about, oh, all of seven minutes.

"Charla, are you going to have any more babies?" she asked. I peered around the stirrups for a sight line of her small head that is cupped by a short, boyish bob. My ob-gyn was teeny tiny. I can't believe she delivers babies without a stepladder. If they made stilt clogs, she would have them. I then stared at the ceiling, trying to think happy thoughts that weren't in the shape of a huge, cold, curved piece of steel. "No," I said with a tightly clenched jaw. "Two is the magic number at our house."

"Well then, have you considered an internist? I'll bet you don't have one. In fact, I'll bet you've been using your annual ob-gyn appointment as a sub for a real physical for a long time."

Wow, a teeny, weeny psychic ob-gyn!

"This will only pinch a bit." She proceeded to go about her job.

I winced and thought happy thoughts, this time about sipping a nice cold glass of Chardonnay while sitting on the porch of an oceanfront beach house and dealing out a hand of cards.

"You know, an internist can give you a breast exam, a pap and a pelvic. Just like me. Plus, she can cover all the other stuff, too. After all, you're nearing forty. It's time you moved on."

Agh. She really is psychic. She knew EXACTLY where to apply the pressure. *You're old. It's time to move on.* Just like that, my ob-gyn put me out to pasture. After two beautiful C-sections, some seriously robust hemorrhoids, and a near bout with gestational diabetes, she moved me along to the Doctors for Aging Women Who Aren't Having Any More Babies. *The Internist.*

She didn't hug me good-bye or give me a pat on the back or offer up a "Thanks for the memories, it was fun." Clearly, she's not from the South. Or else she would have sent me on my way with a casserole and a handwritten note on thick, pastel-pink monogrammed stationery that emphasized that it wasn't my fault. It was her, not me.

I have to admit, I was crushed.

I opened my heart and my uterus to this woman for SIX YEARS, offered up puffy ankles and my very reasonable co-pay, stayed proudly stoic during my sixty-pound weight gain and emergency C-section. And all I got was this.

At the time I feared what seeing an internist meant for the bigger picture. You do know that internists are the "gateway" docs, don't you? They come with a stable of specialty docs—an allergist, a gastroenterologist, a mammographer, an ophthalmologist (Don't need reading glasses just yet? Just wait). The list goes on and on. And do you know how much time is required to look nice and well groomed for that many specialists?

Tripling my medical appointments would start to take its toll. This old car had some mileage on it and the maintenance was about to kill me. Something would have to give in order to better manage my time.

So for me it was ironing, which was just fine with me. I hate ironing. I try desperately to avoid it. I work very hard NOT to iron. Brad dry-cleans his clothes. His overserviced Brooks Brothers shirts eventually disintegrate and *poof*—they literally disappear in a cloud of starchy white cotton. Then I buy him more.

I try to fold the kids' clothes right from the dryer to minimize wrinkles. When they were younger, I had their smocked dresses and john-johns as well as their Strasburg frocks professionally cleaned. And now my kids have nifty dry-weave golf shirts and no-iron button-downs. Which annoys my mother, who thinks somehow I am cheating.

And when it comes to me, I try to buy clothes that don't need to be ironed. I have five knit dresses from one of my favorite women's stores—same style, same size, five different patterns. They. Are. *Awesome.* Honestly, it can be freeing to have a uniform. Kim, my bridge pal, smart and successful business owner and mom of three fabulously well-turned-out daughters, has her own uniform: she wears gorgeous linen tunics that make her look perpetually backlit—all soft and flowy, yet crisp and clean. She always looks thoughtfully pulled together. At one time I aspired to look soft and flowy, yet crisp and clean with a fabulous linen dress from Neiman's—it was a spectacular melon color. Like a good girl, I got it dry-cleaned and pressed every spring. And every season, I put on the dress and took it right off. Put it on and took it right off. I couldn't figure out where to wear it and not end up looking like a piece of wadded-up, coral-colored tissue paper. This dress would be perfect if I didn't have to drive anywhere, sit down anywhere or do anything. Ergo, this beautiful, melon-colored linen dress had no business in my closet and no role in my life. So out with the linen and in with the fabulous, wear-anywhere, stretchy-yet-very-chic shirtdress that I can dial up or down, wear nearly year-round, roll up in a ball and shove in my carry-on luggage, hand-wash and line-dry, wear with a cardigan, dress up with pearls and NEVER, EVER HAVE TO IRON. It's a magic dress, friends. You should get one. Or five.

But some outfits and occasions do call for ironing, and, well, if I truly need to iron, I will. I just hate it. *Because it takes time.* And there is so much other stuff that I have to do when it comes to getting pretty. Plus, I have to set up the ironing board, plug in the iron, and actually do it. And then, I'd do all that work, put on my freshly ironed blouse and realize I didn't quite get that wrinkle ironed out. So sometimes, to shortcut my shortcut, I would iron my clothes after they were on my body.

Do not try this at home. This is a skilled shortcut-to-a-shortcut that takes expertise and dexterity and generally works best when one is wearing knee-to-boob Spanx, aka Kevlar. You just set your iron on warm—not on high, the Kevlar isn't THAT thick—and just slide it gently over the wrinkle. And voilà! But you gotta be careful and remember, your whole body is not wrapped in a Kevlar Spanx. So when you unthinkingly take that iron to press out a slight crease in the collar of that white blouse, it will leave a serious burn. On your right clavicle. That shows.

Last spring I was at a lovely little fund-raising coffee, shoulder to shoulder (or should I say clavicle to clavicle) with a well-dressed, nicely presented volunteer colleague. We stood at the buffet table and she glanced my way, her eyes drawn to my blistered clavicle.

"Ouch," she said. "Straight iron?"

"No," I responded as I reached for a slice of perfectly presented coffee cake carefully arranged on a crystal platter.

"Curling iron?" I shook my head no. She turned to me with a raised brow. I had her full attention now.

"Just a regular iron," I mumbled ungracefully between bites of the incredible coffee cake.

"Really?" she asked with an arched brow. "What happened?"

"I tried to iron a blouse while I was wearing it," I replied, realizing as I said the words out loud how dim-witted I sounded.

She was taken aback but recovered nicely. "Oh, well, it looks like it hurts."

Often, shortcuts do.

Between my job, my husband, my children, my volunteer assignments, friends and never-ending laundry, there is not enough time in the world to do everything that I need to do in one day. And yet getting pretty takes time and, on occasion, ironing.

Is there really a ten-minute beauty plan that can deliver? (Nope.) Are there really only *five* basic clothing items I need to knock 'em dead at work? (Not a chance.) Can I live without Spanx? (It would be like a day without Diet Coke . . . so the answer is *never.*) Can I ever buy anything off the rack that won't need an alteration or two? (Nah.) And so this is why I have

Marine Sergeant Marie, whom I only see when I'm feeling bulletproof, and Rob.

Rob and I met when I was six months pregnant with my
second child. I had a very choppy boy-cut hairstyle that needed
some serious softening up. More than a decade later, Rob is an
indispensable part of my getting-pretty regimen.

"I'm thinking about bangs!"

"No."

"How about *wispy* bangs?"

"No."

"I had a dream I had really long hair that swung around my
shoulders like a Breck girl. Do you ever do extensions?"

"No."

"My hair has a total Julia Roberts *Pretty Woman* vibe when
it's curly! Are perms coming back?"

"No."

"You're mean."

"I'm not mean. I'm saving you from yourself—that's what you
pay me to do. Your hair is too wavy for bangs. 'Wispy'"—insert
air quotes here—"bangs will curl on your forehead like a sau-
sage link. Extensions are cheesy. I will NEVER give a perm in
this salon. Anything else?"

"Um, no."

Instead, Rob turned his considerable talent to my bob. Short
bob. Chin-length bob. Stacked bob. Sassy bob. Dramatic bob.
Rob is the Bob Whisperer. The universe should thank him, write
him a kind note, send him a small token of appreciation. I do it
all the time. No shortcuts when it comes to my tresses. Rob and

I spend LOTS of time together and he regales me with stories of failed shortcuts to pretty. And I sit in pious judgment, too, until he points out my iron burn.

One tale was of a gal who was steered to Rob in a sort of beauty intervention. Apparently, she had hit every salon of note in my Pretty City and had yet to find her hair savior.

"I prefer to wash my hair every three to five days. Oh, and I don't have time to blow it dry or style it," she told Rob. "I need to be able to wash it when I feel like it and then walk out the door."

According to Rob, the Bob Whisperer, he knew it was going to end badly.

"Every few months she would come in and tell me everything that didn't work about her haircut and style," he said. "And you know what? Her hair WAS a wreck. But it wasn't MY doing. There is no magic style that doesn't require a little hair product, a little hot air and a little effort. If she spent half the time she spent complaining about what I couldn't magically do and actually groomed her own head of hair, she'd be amazed."

Rob continued and wisely stated, "I am not a miracle worker. I can't help you if you aren't willing to help yourself." The Bob Whisperer had no tolerance for people like this woman and their inability to take responsibility for their own unconditioned hair condition.

Low maintenance is not the same as no maintenance, and, friends, that is an incredibly important distinction. This woman was too old to have such silly notions. Objects of value, after all, require care, attention and maintenance. Sure, I'd like to maintain a size-six figure while enjoying all the raw cookie dough I can eat, but, alas, it doesn't work like that. I'd like to spend hours tanning in the sun for that bronzed and healthy glow and still have skin as soft as a baby's tush, but it's a no-go. We've got to give ourselves a little help when it comes to looking good and THAT TAKES TIME and good judgment and a reality check. And while we're evaluating possible shortcuts and quick fixes, please remember that there is no shortcut for not trying at all.

Rob once told me about a bedraggled woman schlepping out of Target with her practical "I don't have time to be bothered" haircut and pedestrian flats. Her daughter was a beauty— glammed out in full makeup and hair, along with an artfully casual T-shirt and shorty shorts. She was gabbing on the phone, checking out her reflection in the car window as her mother schlepped two carts of getting-ready-to-head-to-college stuff to the car.

"That mom needed to quit catering to her overindulged daughter and find some time to pull herself together," Rob opined when he shared the story with me while fluffing my wet hair with his hands and looking straight at me. "She looked like she had just given up when it came to her appearance."

I was appalled only because it felt familiar. "Rob, if I ever enter the salon looking like I've thrown in the towel and stopped trying at all, I give you permission to coordinate an intervention immediately."

"That will never happen," he responded calmly while blowing out my hair with his professional Chi dryer.

"How could it NOT happen? You just described my life," I

wailed. "Just look at me, I sit before you in a NAVY CARDIGAN—I'm one step away from middle-aged schlump."

"No, you're not—check out your incredible bob," and he swung my chair around, shoved a big square mirror in my hand and we both openly admired the back of my perfectly stacked head.

Rob loaded me up with product and shooed me out of the salon, as he had other heads to save in his efforts to make the world pretty. And while he sent me into the world with healthy, happy hair, I knew I had walked in the very pedestrian-looking flats of that woman at Target—and more than once. I hadn't just pulled into the HOV lane of getting pretty—looking to nip a few corners of time and energy here and there to get where I was going, I had pulled off the Pretty Interstate completely. It happens to many of us girls every once in a while.

Our cat regularly barfs in the middle of the night somewhere in our house. Despite the frequency of Merlin's messes, I am always mildly surprised by them. It's become a game of sorts in our family. Who can spot the barf first so that they can pretend they never spotted the barf so they don't have to clean up the barf? One day, I bent over Merlin's barf at 6:42 in the morning. By 3:15 that afternoon, I had passed by his little gastrointestinal love offering no less than a dozen times, each time admitting, "Hmm, I really need to clean up the cat barf. But wait, I need to do _____ first."

All told, cat barf is one huge life analogy for me. My days are filled with "I should really [fill in the blank], but *wait*, I need to do [fill in the blank] first!" Often, every minute of every day is spent deciding how to spend it. And while there is no magic formula for getting pretty, there is no doubt that it takes time and intention and, most important of all, I think, experience. It's through that experience that we test shortcuts, check out new pretty products and pretty providers, learn what works and figure out where we're willing to cut corners and where we're not. So while I continue to sidestep Merlin's vomit and hold out hope for a no-burn, body-friendly ironing appliance, I've accepted the fact that I require a three-hour standing date with Rob, the Bob Whisperer, every four weeks; an occasional visit to Marine Sergeant Marie's; and a stable of specialists, and I'll simply just have to find the time to make (most) of it happen.

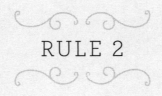

RULE 2

Size Matters

Five years ago on Good Friday, I piled my two children, then seven and nine, in the car to drive ninety miles north of my Pretty City to a nursing home tucked away in a little town called Elkin. My maternal grandmother was ninety-three, and up until a year or so earlier was the picture of health. But a month after my mother and aunt moved her into an assisted-living condo, she fell and broke her hip. It was bizarrely bad timing. Fast-forward six more months, and my grandmother sat in the nursing wing of the same facility, wondering if someone was stealing Mallomars from her minifridge while she was sleeping (which was nearly all the time, so it's entirely possible). It was a swift decline, painful for her two daughters, but possibly not so much for her. One hopes.

My mother called me from the mountains to offer some advice and to prepare me for my visit. "She's really declined, honey. Don't be surprised if she doesn't recognize you." Then she paused to lower her voice: ". . . or the children. Don't take it personally, okay?" My mother and her sister swapped daily the woes of caring for an elderly parent—there are no highs, of course, only lows and lowers as the person you knew morphs into someone you don't.

My grandmother was a force of personality. Through sheer determination and will (and a large dose of her personal faith in Jesus Christ), she weathered a life that while not devastatingly terrible, was not ever, ever easy. It was a drip-drop life of hard work which slowly and ever so gradually eroded her, like water over the rocks in the spring that ran alongside her old house.

When I was young, I visited my grandmother often. We made quarterly trips to see my mother's family and I spent every holiday with them until I married at the ripe old age of thirty-one (that's a lot of holidays). My grandmother was an important, ever-present and unerring extension of my nuclear family. She was the only grandmother I have ever known—blunt, energetic, productive. And I looked like her, too—the same build, the same dark eyes and heavy, hooded eyebrows.

I walked into Room Five at the Hugh Chatham Nursing Center. My grandmother was dressed in a pair of white elastic pants and a yellow sweatshirt with embroidered flowers. Her hair had just been set—it looked like hundreds of little cotton balls had been Velcro'd to her head. She looked right at me with the same brown eyes I had. Hers were a bit milky and rheumy, not the saturated chestnut brown that had dominated our gene pool for generations. Why is it that when people age, some things get bigger (ears, noses, eyebrows) and some get smaller (eyes, teeth, smiles) and color fades? As I was taking her in, I could tell she was doing the same to me.

"Hi, Ma," I offered up as I shuffled my two children into the room and stood before her.

"Well, look at you," she said. "You're not fat."

With that, my ninety-three-year-old grandmother, with her failing mind, failing eyesight and failing temperament, summed up the better part of my then-forty-two-year-old existence. And she did it in only seven words, all of them light, hardly weighing a thing. Easy words, each one a single syllable.

Well, look at you—you're not fat.

My grandmother didn't part with compliments easily. But believe it or not, this was one of them.

My children looked to me, their eyes as large as the cotton-ball curls on my grandmother's head. We did not use the word "fat" in our house. It ranked up there with "stupid" and "duh" and "liar"—language that we simply didn't use. They didn't know that this was my silly little rule, an idiosyncrasy really, to shield my children from potential hurt and confusion (as if that's possible) and from hurting others (as if that's possible either). They don't know yet that in other houses, the little word that packs a big punch is a simple, easy-to-spell adjective that others throw around with abandon.

Other families, of course, have their own words that cannot be spoken. "Four-eyes" or "zit face." For my sister-in-law Elise, she of Irish heritage—it's "pasty." For my friend Suzanne, it's any reference to knock-knees and string beans. For me, it's words like "fat" or "chubby" or "Mindy Cohn."

My grandmother wasn't the first to see me through the lens of weight. It seemed that for all of my life, people had been watching my weight, even when I wasn't. When I was in first grade, I hung out with my next-door neighbor Janine Radar, a small, scraggly girl and the youngest of four children. We would play dolls at her house and glide through the kitchen to sneak cookies into our pockets. I was good at sneaking more than one.

"My mom said I'm not allowed to have as many cookies as you," Janine said one day.

"Why?" I asked, brushing crumbs off my corduroy jumper and breaking open a lemon cream cookie.

"She said I might get pudgy."

"What's 'pudgy'?" I asked.

"Why, Charla!" Janine exclaimed with surprise and a huge smile. "YOU'RE PUDGY." She grinned at me and licked the lemon cream icing, her scrawny legs swinging back and forth.

When you're a kid, discovering you're pudgy, stocky, fat, sturdy or big-boned is a lot like finding out there is no Santa Claus. It comes as a shock the first time you hear it. You've never stopped to consider the idea, much less the alternative. You've never regarded yourself different, apart or unlike before. Suddenly you're aware that others do. Your world is ordered differently after that—from smallest to biggest. And you forever assess where you fit on that continuum.

Like many women, my own weight issues were seeded early. In elementary school, we would sit patiently at our desks and the teacher would call us, one by one, to the front of the room to step on the giant balance-beam scale. She would inch the black weight along the balance beam until it found perfect equilibrium, when it no longer listed in one direction or the other but hung perfectly, silently still. And just for good measure, the teacher let it rest there for a second or two (which seemed like eternity), to make sure that the scale was telling the truth.

Then the teacher would do the unthinkable: she said the number *out loud*, as if to help her remember, and pulled from behind her ear a freshly sharpened, yellow #2 Ticonderoga to write your weight next to your name, where it would be recorded in your permanent school file (which means forever, by the way). Ever since learning I was pudgy, I dreaded this moment of truth every year in elementary school. Much more so than going to the dentist or getting my period in gym class. My cheeks burned. I kept my head down. Only pride kept me from bursting into tears. For me, it was the equivalent of having a scarlet F on my chest. In fifth grade, I was one of the tallest in my class, surpassed only by Sally Churchill and Sandra Zourzoukis. Sally was tall and willowy. Sandra was strong and athletic. I was neither.

There were times when I wasn't pudgy—high school, for example, when I took up a sport and found a boyfriend. And if I recall correctly, a few semesters in college. A year or two postcollege, while living in New York. And a few living in Charlotte—before kids. And now. They are interspersed in my mental time line, like cherries on an ice cream sundae. Looking at life as an ice cream sundae isn't all bad, but it sure seems better with cherries, doesn't it? That's why I don't buy into the idea that weight is just a number. Because this number, just like your SAT test scores, can deeply impact the trajectory of your life.

That's why I (and nearly half of America, I'm convinced) launch into cardiac arrest when getting weighed at the doctor's office. Just ask anyone who wears size-twelve jeans—which, don't forget, is that same half of America. And when I was pregnant? Forget about it. I would step on the scales (again, in the hallway) of my ob-gyn and then get ushered into an exam room where the nurse would take my vitals. "Hmm, your blood pressure is a little elevated, hon," a nurse would say while scribbling in my file.

"Really?" I finally asked one day, launching into what I thought was obvious. "Can I ask you a question? When is it EVER a good idea to take the blood pressure of an extremely pregnant woman who is so puffy she can't wear her own shoes AFTER you have her step on the scales to weigh her IN THE HALLWAY in front of everyone in America . . . or at least everyone who works at Rankin Women's Center!" My face was scarlet with shame—both at the number and at my unseemly outburst. The nurse, in her white clogs and cartoon-riddled nursing smock, cocked her head in sincere contemplation. Truly, it had never occurred to her that a public weighing and a spike in blood pressure could be connected.

My friend Chrissy has an uncanny memory based on her ability to index life milestones by her weight and by whom she was dating or married to at the time. This is an especially amazing feat as Chrissy's weight (like mine) not only fluctuated quite a bit over the years, but she also dated and married a lot. "Don't you remember, Char? That was when I was dating Larry and I was so skinny, had short, permed hair and wore that awesome emerald-green dress that made my boobs look big?" Actually, when she framed it up that way, I did remember.

Unlike Chrissy, I had never indexed a life moment based on weight until 9/11. At the time I was home with a ten-week-old baby. Slumped semicatatonic on my sofa, sporting days-old sweats, unwashed hair and raw breasts, I watched images of the planes slamming into the towers seemingly on a continuous loop. Smoke pouring, people running, people jumping, people dying. I heard first-person accounts from my friends on how they evacuated nearby buildings, got off the island, connected with spouses. I was horrified and transfixed. I heard stories about women shedding heels, dumping uncomfortable clothes, getting down to the basics so they could get to safety. Suddenly everyone was talking about a plan, a safe house, a bag with batteries, bottled water, canned food, face masks and Cipro. I fretted about my young family's fate and safety.

I played out all the scenarios about moving everyone to a safe place. Creating a meeting spot for extended family. Getting out of a major metropolitan city to a smaller, less crowded one. Getting out of our house. Getting my child out of our house—breaking a window, tossing him to safety.

That's when I realized that my big, puffed-up, recently-given-birth rear end could not fit out of anything but the big, roomy front door. Not a first-story picture window, and certainly not a second-story bedroom window. If disaster hit my house and the front door was not an exit option, I was doomed. I was too wide.

For the first time, it occurred to me that my weight had less to do with vanity and more to do with managing my family. Getting them out of a dangerous situation. Picking one up and running like the wind. There was no camouflaging that fact with a billowing blouse in a nice, soft teal color . . . I couldn't do it.

In a crisis, I could not save my children. Dramatic? Of course. True? Ditto.

I cried at the realization that my weight wasn't getting in the way of my dreams (which is so cliché), but in the way of my life (which is so real and sadly practical).

To feel better, I ate some macaroni and cheese. Carbs always make things better.

Like it or not, weight can be a defining factor in who we are and what we become. I long ago realized that carrying extra weight is like losing one of your five senses—it heightens all the others. So in addition to my incredible sense of smell, I have an amplified sense of humor, an intensified ability to see the absurd and an above-average ability to laugh at myself (and, admittedly, on many occasions, at others). In the absence of skinny, one must compensate, it seems. And like most of my husky sisters, I did just that—developing a wit that not only allowed me to survive the trauma of all things adolescent, but also occasionally to thrive. I was the funny girl with the sharp tongue who stayed on high alert when it came to catty girls and obnoxious boys.

The greater your sins of poundage, the less, it seems, you matter. Want to have a significant presence in this world? Present as a waif. This inverse correlation is odd. There is unspoken respect for small and skinny, no matter how frightfully frail. If we comment on someone who is overweight—there is communal acknowledgment. "Hmm, yes, poor thing, she really does need to lose some weight." No one disagrees on too much weight. But commenting on someone who is thin, skinny, small is considered sour grapes, a sort of professional jealousy that seems unbecoming of us bigger girls.

In fact, no one comments on the skinny girl save to compliment and wonder aloud, "How does she do it?" Skinny speaks of restraint, discipline, self-control. Some of us might never admit it aloud, but there is inherent goodness in skinny. We all aspire to skinny. Who in the world aspires to fat? Fat is so inappropriate—it's slovenly, chaotic, unbecoming.

The only girls who talk about weight are the girls who don't have a weight problem. How they need to lose those last five pounds of baby weight, those last five pounds from family vacation in the Turks, those last five pounds of BLAH BLAH BLAH. And then their friends, the lovely and supportive friends they are, chirp in with sweet assurances that they don't need to lose a pound, that those pounds aren't noticeable at all in those cute, hip-hugging jeans, but if they're serious, have they thought about juicing?

Sturdy girls don't bring up weight in group settings—why make everyone feel uncomfortable by pointing out the obvious? "Hmm, I really need to lose those fifty pounds I gained over the last five years. I mean, between kids, my job, keeping up the house and visiting my best friends, Mrs. Shubert and Aunt Jemima, it just snuck up on me. I don't understand it. Are you going to finish those fries?" And your friends, being the lovely and supportive friends they are, can't very well agree with you OUT LOUD. So discussions about the weight-afflicted are off-limits and instead we talk about hair—because none of my girl-friends are bald and we can all contribute something to that conversation.

Even now I have this tiny twinge, an ever-so-slight pull in my chest when my children get weighed at their annual checkups, the thought that they are a pound or two away from getting judged on something besides their fantastic sense of humor or ability to craft the perfect spitball. Like my heinous classroom scale nightmare, the scales at the pediatrician are situated in the *hallway*—where EVERYONE CAN SEE! It's so public, so out there for everyone to judge. Weight is a private matter—much like one's salary—it's unseemly to discuss the numbers.

But here's the irony about weight—while it might be inappropriate to discuss one's (heavy) weight, you can't really hide it like you can other things. It's possible to hide the wine bottles in the laundry hamper, the ashtray under the couch and even the "happy pills" in your underwear drawer. But you can't hide fifty pounds, especially if you have no idea how much space fifty pounds takes.

I know this because I am the poster child for the spatially challenged. I hate jigsaw puzzles because I just don't see how those pieces all fit together. And I go through about half a dozen Tupperware containers daily trying to find the right fit for my leftovers.

One day, Brad watched, frozen in anthropological shock, as I tried to fit spaghetti into a plastic container. Spaghetti spilled out of the top and down the sides. "You didn't possibly believe that four cups of pasta would fit into that eight-ounce container, did you?" he asked.

"No, I'm doing this for comic relief," I answered tartly as I squished down meatballs and sauce with a wooden spoon. "Of course I thought the spaghetti would fit."

"Is that why there is an inch of leftover soup swirling around in a five-gallon tub in the fridge?" he countered. I gave him the stink eye and sopped up the red sauce that was pooling across the counter like a bloodstain.

This might explain my extreme spatial confusion when I lost a load of weight. Certainly my scales told a story. My clothes echoed the lovely little tale by winnowing down six dress sizes. My nine-year-old's hands could finally clasp together around my waist in a hug. But the reality was this: I had no idea how much ROOM I'd taken up in this world weighing in at two hundred pounds. And conversely, I had no idea how much LESS room I took up minus sixty. My spatial handicap blinded me to the obvious. While I *knew* I was a "touch" overweight, I had no spatial understanding of what that meant. I didn't seem to take up more than my fair share of room on the sofa. I fit just fine in the seats in the movie theater. I just barely didn't have to shop at the "special stores." Sure I broke my girlfriend's wicker patio chair, but I was eight months pregnant, and she was a lovely sport about it. So for about a year, I was still getting my bearings even as I continued to lose the weight. And despite my spatial challenges, it was all coming together.

I felt better, I moved faster, I was stronger. All told, getting rid of unnecessary weight made me bionic (except I wasn't a promising tennis pro with fabulous hair who nearly died in a freak skydiving accident). Lugging around all that weight like a Sherpa at Base Camp didn't seem like a big deal until I realized how high I could really go. So I don't buy these lame arguments that big is beautiful and we should embrace XXXXLs, and that people are perfectly happy and content and fabulous carrying around extra poundage. Because it's not true. They might tell you it's true, they might *want* it to be true, but it's a lie. While you don't want to be too skinny (there is likely some emotional baggage getting lugged around if you are), neither do you want too much pudge. It might not make you miserable, but it's unwieldy, both on your frame and on your emotional state. Pudge gets in the way, it's inconvenient, it's tiresome. And for anyone who wants to yell at me for making politically incorrect comments about *F-A-T*, then may I remind you, I've been there . . . so I can.

Last spring, I remember meeting a lovely woman from California when she was visiting friends in Charlotte. We ended up seated next to each other, poolside, at an intimate dinner party, hosted by a power couple as part of an art museum fund-raiser. Like our hostess, my dinner companion was an interior designer. She was also fun, thoughtful, interesting. My kind of gal.

We talked about kids, husbands, working moms, our faith and finally tripped onto the subject of weight and the enormous pressure of California "thin." This was a very smart, very pretty and very well-put-together size four. Which, apparently by L.A. standards, was on the high end of the scale.

"My weight fluctuates about five pounds. I would spend incredible amounts of time and energy losing that five pounds. Gain it back and then spend incredible amounts of time and energy losing that five pounds again. But what it took me some time to realize was that I was happier, more mellow and a better mom and wife WITH the five pounds." And likely less hungry, too, I imagined.

Losing that five pounds and keeping it off dominated her emotional landscape. It wasn't obvious, but if she paid attention, the telltale signs were there—she was less bionic.

Size mattered. Ironically, she had to be okay with those extra five pounds to find her perfect emotional weight. And I had to lose sixty pounds to find mine.

A year following the *Oprah* debacle, when my family and I did our requisite two weeks in June in the mountains with my parents, my brother and his family, I had a moment. This was during the year of some hard personal work—a new eating *regimen* ("D-I-E-T" is another word we don't use in my house) and a new walking schedule. I had decided to embark on a low-carb, low-fat "weight-management program" (no D-I-E-T for me, remember) that involved sweating more and eating better than I had in a long, long time. Besides the constant fear that I might never poop again (low-carb "weight-management programs" will do that, you know), I was losing the weight that had shown up on television like some specter.

My hard work paid off when on a Friday night in July, I was

able to fit into a dress that I had worn only in my middle-aged dreams—a chic wraparound garment in white linen (yes, a dress that needed ironing, but hey, I was on vacation and had downtime). For sturdy girls, wraparound dresses can be tricky—too much material can add a lot of bulk. And white? Well, law! Everyone knows big girls should *not* wear white. Piped in black with classic peaked lapels and a tightly cinched sash, the dress had one more incredible quality. *It was sleeveless*. I could not honestly recall the last time I'd worn a sleeveless dress. Even my wedding dress had sleeves. I had long ago learned that sleeveless "is not my friend," to quote my mother. But now? Now sleeveless and Charla were besties.

I wrapped myself in that smart linen dress purchased at Neiman's Last Call outlet in Austin during a girls' weekend with some of my other besties and I stared in the mirror. Not because I was smitten with my image, but because I was stunned by the incongruity of it. *This wasn't, this couldn't be, me.* Despite the exercise, the diet, the sweat—it didn't seem real. I was spatially confused, remember, so it took a moment to compute.

But once I took in the image in the mirror, it was, I have to say, a stellar personal moment. No, it did not trump the birth of my two children, or getting hired for my first job, or getting asked for my hand in marriage by a really swell guy whose green eyes made me swoon. But still, it was a moment, and it was mine.

As I floated down the stairs feeling like a forty-plus-year-old, part-time-working, full-time-married-with-two-kids Princess Mom, my mother was standing at the bottom wiping her hands on a dishcloth. She glanced up at me casually. "Why are you wearing *that*? Don't waste that outfit on tonight—save it for something special. You're *entirely* overdressed." And with that, she turned and walked away.

I had no words.

For the love of Jenny Craig, this was a CHIC, WHITE, SLEEVELESS WRAPAROUND LINEN DRESS WITH PEAKED LAPELS PURCHASED FOR A DEAL AT NEI-MAN'S LAST CALL! And what could be more special than the enormous relief of knowing that I wasn't destined—if but for tonight—to a life sentence as Middle-Aged Frumpy Mom with a Wry Sense of Humor and a Keen Nose for a Good Sale? How could she not see that?

I can't explain it and I'm not proud of it, but right then I had a very unnattractive adolescent moment. I turned around, stomped upstairs to my room and ripped off the dress to put on "regular" clothes, feeling like a chastised teenager. An unattract-ive, misunderstood chastised teenager. I slammed around my room and tried to explain it all to my sister-in-law, an obvious outsider to my family's version of Appearance Dysfunction, who had knocked on the bedroom door I had just dramatically slammed shut. She listened to me vent, O she of red hair and alabaster skin and gorgeous legs, and then quietly picked up the chic, white, sleeveless, wraparound linen dress with peaked lapels heaped in a ball on the floor (looking like I felt) and handed it back to me.

"You look fantastic in this dress. Now put it on, fix your makeup and let's go," she said.

And just like that, my little preteen temper tantrum ended.

I sucked it up, wrapped myself back in that white wraparound dress and walked out of the house, past my mother, without a word. Both of us wondering what had just happened.

But I knew. It was this: I was forty-two years old and I had, for the first time in a long while, felt pretty. Not "I'm the prettiest girl in the room" pretty—that mantle is not available and not necessary to me. But also not "fourth-runner-up pretty" as in "at least I have good hair and my teeth haven't shifted that much." Or "Wow, this skirt makes my size-fourteen tush look like a size twelve." I had gone from just barely adequate to above-average presentable.

It wasn't ego. It was relief, mixed with a little bit of panic. I wanted to enjoy the feeling, because who knew how long it would last?

My mother, whom I love with all my heart and who is my biggest fan, didn't intend to deprive me of that moment. It was quite accidental—the deepest wounds often are. But after our forty-two-year relationship and best efforts, we're still bruising those same tender spots.

It slowly dawned on my mother that her casual comment had unintended consequences drummed up from four decades of Appearance Anxiety. I called her from dinner with a teary apology, which she graciously accepted. After all, she was babysitting our kids that night.

And I know despite my best intentions that I will likely one day do the same thing to my own daughter—accidentally derail her turn to shine, to feel pretty. Perhaps mothers do it unknowingly because they know their children will have more than one moment. They have enough life experience to know that possibilities and shining moments and dreams are much bigger than "pretty" or "cute" or "thin." I want my daughter to see that moments, like people, come in all shapes and sizes and that while some occasionally might fall under the "pretty" banner, many don't.

It sometimes feels treasonous and wrong, but I'm an expat of pudge and I never want to return to my former country, the land of the Chubby and Cheery. Because no matter how hard I tried—and believe me, I have tried—wit and good humor will never, ever outweigh the feeling of a chic, white, sleeveless, wraparound linen dress with peaked lapels purchased for a deal at Neiman's Last Call. Never, ever, *ever*, you hear me?

Sometimes getting pretty can be a means to an end. "When I lose weight, get new boobs, go blond, get a nose job, [insert your beauty dilemma here], I will get more dates, more interesting friends, a better job, invitations to the best parties, a cuter house, apartment, lake cabin, [insert your dream here]." In other words, getting pretty can hold the promise of a better life.

But there I was, with no aspirations that hinged on my appearance. For the first time, I had no endgame—I had lost the weight that had for so long held me back. Changing my appearance now wouldn't significantly alter my life. I wasn't going to give my husband intimacy every day for a year. Been there.

Done that. It wouldn't make me any happier or more fulfilled or more productive as a wife, employee, mother and daughter. Would it?

This was new territory, I must admit, a long way from my college days when I figured out weight-loss equations during statistics class. *Three pounds a week times eight weeks equals twenty-four pounds equals the dress I bought that I can't currently zip but hope to wear to Spring Formal, which I don't have a date to yet but we'll worry about that later because once I lose twenty-five pounds the guys at the PKA house are gonna be lining up . . . Where are my Coke and M&M's and when is that geology exam again . . . and I have to make an appointment for a spiral perm.*

(Did I mention I flunked statistics? I'm terrible at math.)

There is a legacy to weight and perceptions of it, of course. One woman's quest for skinny translates to a daughter's woes of poundage. My mother, while never heavy, gingerly managed her weight, aware of the scale and even more aware of her mother's opinion of it. Therefore, she pulled back on her opinion of mine. But I could see it and sense it. Her hyperintuitive maternal awareness of my weight revealed itself in her eyes, in her delicate approach to shopping for my clothes, in the words not said when I had second helpings. She knew me too well to know that living in the country of the Chubby and Cheery was hardly fun. She was trying to help, of course. Her deliberate quietness on the subject made me feel loved, but no less chunky.

Now as a parent, I'm doing the same.

A few years ago my daughter asked me, "Mom, do I need a diet?" She was in the third grade and perched on a stool in our kitchen, enjoying some creative and well-balanced snack lovingly prepared by her fabulous mother.

There was a silence so great and so thick, it felt like sludge. First of all, where did she learn about the Word That Shall NOT Be Spoken? And second, my offspring is the most perfectly created creature on the planet, except when she is not. She doesn't need a D-I-E-T.

"Why? Did someone tell you you needed to go on a diet?" I tried to sound nonchalant while quickly rolling through my mental Rolodex to find the nasty, insensitive and clueless person who introduced my daughter to the D-I-E-T word and didn't have the decency to teach her its grammatically correct usage.

"Well, no," she admitted as her little hand hovered over a whole-grain graham cracker swathed in peanut butter, topped with a banana slice and decorated with one semi-sweet chocolate chip. "But Grandma was talking about her diet the other day, and I wondered if I should have one, too."

Ha, I should have KNOWN! My own flesh and blood betrayed me (again). *Take your time. Think*, I thought to myself. Obviously this was a pivotal moment in the life of my daughter, and her entire self-image hinged on my incredibly healthy and well-delivered response. But then I thought to myself, *I'm her mother and that's what we do, we accidentally screw up and send our children into years of therapy.* (Right?) So I changed tacks and simply tried to neutralize the situation, not try to be some Oprah-like mom-hero from some Oxygen movie who says exactly the right thing at exactly the right moment. I mean, who are those people anyway and do we even like them?

"Well, if you know how to make smart food choices and know all about healthy foods, you don't really have to worry about having a diet. And you know how to do that."

"Oh, does that mean Grandma makes bad food choices?" asked sweet daughter as she peeled apart a skim-milk cheese stick. A satisfied smile spread slowly across my face. Aha— chance to flip the mater tables a little. It was a sweet victory, as tasty as Ben & Jerry's New York Super Fudge Chunk ice cream.

"Why yes, it does, honey," I replied with more than a little bit of satisfaction, popping a few chocolate chips into my mouth. "Grandma. Makes. Very. Bad. Food. Choices. Be sure to ask her about that, okay? In fact, why don't I dial her up right now—I'm sure she's home—and you two can discuss all the bad food choices she has made over the years."

Wow, that was easier that I imagined. I high-fived my imaginary friends, Ben and Jerry, in honor of this small but important victory. And I debated whether to apologize to my mother for throwing her under the ice cream truck. Of course, my mother emerged from this freak accident unscathed and with her reputation as "Grandmother of the Decade" fully intact. And so did my daughter. Because neither was wound nearly as tight as I when it came to getting or needing a D-I-E-T.

Years later, I went bikini shopping with my daughter. Not for me, but for her. She was by then a middle schooler, and in a flash-fry of a second she'd sprouted long legs, long thick wavy hair the color of chestnuts, curves and all the accoutrements (in other words, an alien gave birth to her, as she was clearly nothing like me). But behind those hazel-green eyes and newly straightened teeth was the sweet girl who doodled hearts and flowers around her name, occasionally visited her favorite stuffed animals that sat in a basket in the far corner of her room and called me "Mommy" often enough to remind me of her inherent sweetness.

She asked if we could go together to try on bikinis, and so we did. At Belk, we grabbed nearly a dozen tops and as many complementary bottoms and headed into the dressing room. I'm probably telling you something you already know, but these days they sell bathing suits in parts. You can literally mix and match the tops and bottoms—instead of Garanimals, it's really a Gara-kini. I found this fascinating and, as a marketer, brilliant. After all, men's suits have been sold separately for years; hence the ubiquitous sport coat. Even the Middle-Aged Mom Bathing Classic—the Skirted Tankini—comes in parts these days. Of course, all of this was lost on me as I have NEVER purchased a bathing suit in more than one part unless it was a matching muumuu to cover my very conservative one-piece.

One might think I considered this a bonding moment with my daughter, but I didn't. That I waxed nostalgic with her about my own bathing-suit shopping trips with my own mother to the same department store. Nope. That I recalled with fondness how my mother and I would stroll through the aisles of Belk, arms linked, swapping affectionate repartee. None of that either.

For my mother, shopping with me was like an act of war. She

took Sun Tzu's thirteen tactics to heart as she prepared to go shopping with her petulant, chunky, four-eyed, braces-faced daughter. I wasn't at war with my mother as much as I was at war with all I couldn't be. And in those poorly lit dressing rooms, all of my flaws were brought to light and I had nowhere to vent my frustration save on her.

But if my mother is anything, she is tenacious, and years later she finally realized that victory lay in situational positioning and did what she should have done years earlier—she left me at home. And brought gads of bathing suits (and all other forms of clothing) home to me. I would arrive from school and find stacks of bathing suits, cover-ups and shorts sitting on my bed. We had a tacit understanding—I knew what to do and she knew I would call her if I needed her. Strangely, I did call her because I did need her. Despite the tears of anger and frustration, I still yearned for loving reassurance and firm guidance as I sorted through clothes styled for "girls like me" and prayed that something would work.

Even later, when bathing-suit shopping wasn't as bad as a root canal without novocain, I appreciated NOT having to endure the fluorescent lights, the three-way mirror and nosy salesclerks. Since then, I have purchased nearly all of my bathing suits online. And prior to that, over the phone. (Remember when you would go through a catalog and then call a number on the phone and speak to a real person and tell them all the stuff you wanted to order and then they would send it to you? Crazy, huh?)

Despite her assets, my tall, thin, long-legged and boobalicious best pal, Suzanne, treats bathing-suit shopping the same way. I've known Suzanne since college, and while she lives in New Jersey and I live in the southern part of heaven, we chat, e-mail and text regularly, see each other often and generally stay entrenched in each other's life and corresponding beauty dramas. Which is ironic, really, as we are a bit like Abbott and Costello and our fashion challenges could not be more different.

Suzanne recently ordered five suits online from different stores. They all came—some tankinis with bikini bottoms, some bikini tops with high-waisted bottoms (apparently, it looked good on the model, so Suzanne thought to give it a try) and of course, the dreaded skirted tankini.

"My husband is getting ready for work. My kids are buzzing around. And I'm trying on bathing suits," Suzanne relayed to me. In fact, we scheduled time so she could recount the entire ordeal, it was that rough. "I tried on a dozen different combinations with zero response from anyone. I felt totally ignored. They thought they were being nice."

Finally Suzanne put on the last combination (a full-coverage, sleeved tankini top with a skirted bottom) and stood in front of the mirror. Then she walked over to her husband and oldest child, who both screamed in happy unison, "Yeah, that's the one!"

"Really?" Suzanne told me later. "I looked like I was heading to a tennis tournament—completely covered on the top and nary an inch of thigh showing on the bottom. The family consensus was that Mom looked great in a bathing suit that showed my neck, face and knees and nothing else."

It was a sobering moment, for sure. "My family liked me best in a Lycra habit," concluded my lapsed Catholic BFF.

Nowadays Suzanne focuses on buying shoes—fabulous sandals, trendy flip-flops, the perfect wedge. And she didn't waste all that fashion-forward footwear on bathing suits—that summer she decided to wear shorts and a cute T or a flattering Athleta halter dress to the pool.

"I saved time, money and angst and I'm SPF-protected!" she proudly stated. She'd found peace.

So my daughter had no idea that I (and apparently most forty-something moms across the hemisphere) hadn't tried on a bathing suit in a dressing room of a department store (or any retail outlet for that matter) in the last twenty-five years. That's a long time and a lotta bathing suits.

I sat down and started managing the trying-on, taking-off process and it occurred to me that I was having that Every Mom moment of sitting tirelessly in a changing room, hanging up item after item after item on those flimsy little plastic hangers while my child flung item after item after item on the floor. It was a thankless job, just as my mother lamented all those years ago at the exact same department store. But I did reflect that I was hanging up TWICE the items with all these bikini parts. One-piece bathing suits are not only modest, but also less work. My mother should thank me.

And while I found myself thinking about my mother, I noted that there was a profound difference between my experience and hers. First, I was sitting in a dressing room with a child who was reasonably well adjusted and emotionally balanced (for now). She was also appropriately appreciative and generally pleasant (for now). I felt a stab of guilt and remorse as I recalled my unbearably boorish behavior toward my mom and put another check on the list of all the reasons why I love her.

Second, and I fully own this, I was over-the-moon happy that my daughter could not just wear a bikini, but looked good in it. You might think it was parental hubris, maternal self-indulgence or just my own weird stuff, and perhaps it was all that and more. But there was so much more tangled up in that mother-daughter hairball. Simply put, I found great joy in the fact that my daughter could look in the mirror unfettered by any emotional and physical baggage and like what she saw. Of course, to tell her any of this would have given the moment more energy than it deserved. Because I know at the end of the day, it's not about rocking it in a bikini but feeling great in your own skin.

And you can only feel great in your own skin when you're comfortable with your shape and weight. The reality is that size does matter. It can interfere with our ability to know our true self. Because we are so much more than others choose to see from the outside—the number on a scale, a gorgeous white linen dress, or a perfect tankini. And sometimes we accidentally back into a category that defines—and later constrains—us. And our size—too big or too small—can hold us back from the incredible and life-changing opportunity to figure it out ourselves.

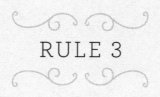

RULE 3

First Impressions
(and Annuals)
Count

To admit the power of first impressions unnerves us. It's likely because we all have a story or two (or many) of disastrous first impressions, which only reinforces their significance. And while we're wired with a predilection for second chances and do-overs, deep down we all know that nothing compares to that first-time moment. We hate how much such moments matter in large part because we know how much they do. And part of the power of first impressions is that while we can control them, we can't control them all the time.

Which is why I felt compelled to help my friend Lizzie. She and I met more than a decade ago when she interviewed for a job at my firm in Charlotte. We hit it off and became fast friends. Lizzie is Jewish by way of Columbia University, and her husband, Will, is a lapsed New York City Catholic by way of Harvard. Lizzie kept her maiden name, Will kept his maiden name, and they saddled their son with some hyphenated pack mule of a name. They are funny, smart and irreverent and treated living in Charlotte as some sort of curious little social experiment. And, of course, I did what I could to help, as if they needed any.

We were at the beach for the weekend, both families sharing a beach house and enjoying the mildly frenetic spring weather. We discussed their son's recent acceptance by one of Pretty City's outstanding private schools. They were pleased, of course, as John was a very bright, rising kindergartner and the school would be a good fit.

"Well, before you all start school," I began, opening a bottle of wine to celebrate (because when your firstborn starts kindergarten, the entire freakin' family starts school), "you need to figure something out. Lizzie, you either need to change your name to match Will's, or you need to wear your wedding band."

Lizzie looked at me, her interest piqued. Will, possibly the smartest guy I hang out with on a regular basis, stared at me blankly.

"Look," I continued. "You each have a different last name. Lizzie doesn't wear a wedding ring, and when she does, it doesn't really look like a wedding ring—it's some cloisonné number, pretty, but not a traditional wedding set, okay? People are gonna assume, 'cuz that's what people do, that John's parents are divorced and that Will is remarried and that Lizzie is not, hence the naked left. So at every parent meeting, they'll rubberneck, trying to spot the 'new wife,' wagering if everyone 'gets along.'"

"Naked what?" asked Will, working to backtrack.

"Naked left. She has a naked left hand!" How could the smartest guy I know not keep up? "If you're married and you're a guy and you don't wear a wedding band, everyone thinks you're a cad. If you're married and you're a girl and you don't wear a wedding band, everyone assumes you're not married. It just doesn't compute. *No comprendo, amigo.* In the absence of information, people will fill in the blanks themselves."

"Wow, that's a lot of work. Why don't people just ask?" Will wondered.

I sighed dramatically—this was like explaining rain to a bedouin.

"They're never going to ask—that would be rude. Inappropriate. Nosy. Instead, they're going to draw wildly inaccurate and presumptuous conclusions about you and your family based on the information they have, which is kinda thin. I'm sorry if those of us in this neck of the woods are not as enlightened as the rest of the world on all these hybrid and hyphenated last names, but that's my take on it."

I was on a Chardonnay roll. They needed to back away. I needed room.

"Is that how you want to launch the next thirteen years of your social life at this lovely school—confusing others, making them pause and ask themselves, 'Are they together? Are they divorced? Do they live together? Do I acknowledge any of this? Will it be awkward? Will I say anything wrong? Maybe I'll just walk the other way.'"

I paused to pour myself another glass of wine. (Okay, I might have poured a third glass of wine.) But I spoke the truth. For better or for worse, the attempt to make order of the chaos of our lives dictates that we make assumptions and draw conclusions—often quickly and without all the required information. Which only proves my point—first impressions provide important details in how others determine where they (and you) fit in. Sadly, this has little to do with the person making the impression, and everything to do with the person forming it.

This is why what you wear on the first day of school is so cataclysmically important.

My first day at private middle school could only be described as one of the seven levels of Purgatory (not Dante's Hell, but Purgatory was bad enough). I had matriculated semisuccessfully in our local public schools and wasn't remotely interested in a new school where a small band of kids had been in the same class since kindergarten. And of course, I didn't want to transfer to a school with a dress code (not uniforms, but a dress code). And I certainly had no interest or skill in cracking the social code of a new coterie of girls whose reputation suggested that they penned a book called *How to Humiliate the New Girl in Seven Days or Less*. But bad grades and some poor choices in friends had forced my parents' hand, and they meant business.

While I knew one or two of the girls from a distance, I didn't know any of them well enough to throw myself at their mercy and beg for social leniency. I did, however, know a few of the boys.

The Johnson twins were identical twins who lived down the street from me and in some way, shape or form played a starring role in nearly any trouble I EVER brought upon myself. That said twins were also in attendance at said private school where my parents thought I would receive calming guidance from well-adjusted, well-reared youths and challenging instruction from upstanding, well-educated teachers, was rich.

I know identical twins are, well, identical. But these two were bizarrely indistinguishable. They didn't have to work at all to confuse and annoy adults with their extreme "twin-ness." That would have been too gratuitous and too easy, and they were far too clever and daring to bank on something as obviously redundant as their shared DNA. Their most powerful tool was a different kind of shared duality—their ability to so surefootedly walk the line between using their powers for good and using them for evil. And the Johnson twins took it to a level of epic proportions. Even I, one of a few who witnessed up close, personal and in Technicolor their effortless transition from charming and genuinely good to hair-raising, juvie-hall evil, had a hard time discerning their strategy.

Good or evil. Good or evil. Good or evil. It kept a girl on her toes, that's for sure.

"What's got you so keyed up?" one of the twins asked a few days before school started. Apparently, my keen sense of adventure and appetite for prepubescent danger had dulled a bit as summer waned and my pending social doom approached.

I ran through a list in my head. What DIDN'T have me keyed up about changing schools in that gawky, awkward stage of pimpled adolescence? I rolled through a few dozen of the worries that were keeping me up at night and finally found one that didn't seem too pathetic, but still very real.

"I don't know what to wear," I said. "It's the first day of school and I need to wear something that makes me fit in." Which is girl code for "I need to wear something that doesn't make me stick out." As if that could ever really happen, but a chubby gal with newly minted contact lenses can dream that the first impression she will make will be nothing short of dazzling, can't she?

"That's easy," a Johnson twin announced. "I can help you figure out what to wear on the first day of school."

I looked at him suspiciously. After all, this wasn't my first Doublemint Twins rodeo. I narrowed my eyes and sized him up in silence. Good or evil. Good or evil. Good or evil?

He looked at me, shrugged his shoulders and ran out to the yard to chase down my little brother and drop him on his head. Definitely using his powers for good, I concluded as I followed him.

Later, the same Johnson twin (I think) came to my house and in a brisk, efficient manner helped me pick out my first-day-of-school outfit. The fact that he was unfazed by the whole thing gave me a modicum of confidence and I relaxed a bit. Plus, I bore witness to a Johnson twin using his powers for good—namely, helping a pal nail an important first impression. It was a rare sight indeed.

And I remember that first day, walking into the classroom, down the middle aisle, to take my seat, living out every *Afterschool Special* cliché ever written. There was Cindy in her green A-line skirt and white blouse with the Peter Pan collar piped in the same kelly green. There was Karen, the athlete, looking relaxed and cute in a loose and comfortable Laura Ashley dress.

And there was Lisa with her Pappagallo wedges that matched her outfit to perfection.

As I made my way to my desk and stole glances up and down each aisle, a sinking feeling set in. I realized that I did fit in with my khaki A-line skirt, blue chambray button-down shirt, canvas belt and Bass Weejuns. I just fit in with the wrong gender. My identical-twin frenemy had dressed me the only way he knew how—he picked out what HE would wear on the first day of school. Evidence that he was indeed using his powers for good. But it was a social death knell for me. The only thing I was missing was a tie and a navy blazer.

There were many things that set the precedent for that humiliating year of personal growth, but surely that first-impression fashion fiasco contributed to a downward spiral that stretched through 180 grueling days that culminated in the moving-up ceremony and the end-of-year dance.

Our moving-up ceremony included a performance of "Come Sail Away" featuring yours truly on the flute. If the flute and a song by the band Styx seem a bit at odds to you, let me assure they were. But my three years in "band" made me a bit of a musical novelty at a school that had no music program. So I played my flute at all manner of special events and assemblies, simply reinforcing my starring role as perpetual outsider and stark, raving nerd. Even winning the headmaster's quarterly award—E Pluribus Unum—drove home the point. It was Latin for "out of many, one."

Yep, that was me all right. Out of many, I was the one girl

who couldn't land a date to the end-of-the-year dance. The theme was "Stairway to Heaven" and the Johnson twins had dates—one asked the sporty cute girl. The other asked the other sporty cute girl who went to another school. Which, by the way, I think is incredibly poor form. Asking girls from another school to the prom when there is available inventory at your own school smacked of confidence and popularity—and I hated it. My class was pairing up like the floods were coming and this was the last dance before the Ark sailed away.

I wasn't entirely surprised I didn't have a date, but ever the perpetual optimist, I held out hope that there would be some break in the time-space continuum and some hunky, athletic boy would step into my path and all but BEG me to attend the prom with him.

Instead, meet Raymond Reynolds. Raymond was about three inches shorter than I, with a weirdly unsettling sense of humor and dishwater-brown hair. Raymond wasn't a bad guy, but he was about as far down on the social food chain as one flute-playing gal who dressed like a boy on her first day of school.

Raymond approached me one afternoon at the end of the day with what I can only describe as a bit of a swagger—as if a stubby, slightly unathletic boy can even master a swagger.

"Charla, I'm thinking you might want to go the dance with me." That's exactly how he put it, I do not lie. This proved the adage that short, nebby, obnoxious men likely started out as short, nebby, obnoxious boys.

I just stared at him. He had this slightly stiff but smug look in his eyes. I tried to put my finger on why Raymond looked like a slightly puffed-up dishwater-brown peacock. So I stared at him some more. Then it dawned on me.

Raymond Reynolds knew I would say yes.

Not because he was a really neat guy with a swell personality and an athletic frame that topped out at more than five feet. He knew it was a sure thing because he was sure he'd be my only choice. He was confident because of my lack of offers, not because his offer was all that appealing.

Raymond didn't want to go to the dance with me any more than I wanted to go to the dance with him. Even at that age I recognized his desperation, and I didn't want it rubbing off on me. I had enough problems.

"No thanks, Raymond," I said, in a rare moment of clarity, and turned to walk away.

He blinked a few times, appeared a bit shocked and shook his head as if to shake free some earwax. He was shocked that the goofy new girl who made the abysmal impression on the first day of school and had a yen for woodwinds had the audacity to decline such a generous offer. "What do you mean 'no thanks'?" he demanded as he walked along behind me. "Who are you going to go with? Who in the world is going to ask *you*?"

He was agitated and looking around. That's when I noticed that he had a group of boys watching him, coaching him and prodding him along. Including, of course, the infamous Johnson twins, who were PRETENDING to use their powers for good but likely hoping to collect cash from the bets they wagered on this mortifying exchange. An exchange that even I would bet money they orchestrated.

"Um, I'm not sure who I'm going to go with, but I don't think I'm going with you. Thanks anyway," I responded as I walked toward the door, away from Raymond, the boy who fancied himself my only hope for a prom date.

"They told me you'd say yes!" he shouted as a last-minute Hail Mary while his humiliation sank in. The humiliation of getting rejected by the nerdy, desperate girl who was supposed to yes.

My cheeks flamed. I kept my head down and headed home. I didn't mention the incident to anyone. The Johnson twins, who certainly had a modicum of self-preservation, didn't bring it up either. In the meantime, I pushed it all to the back of my mind and headed home to practice my scales, in heady preparation for another painful flute accompaniment.

Later that month, I was at my friend Chrissy's house. Chrissy was a year older, a decade more mature and personified all things trendy and current. We were friends because our mothers were friends. Which meant that my lack of social standing at school didn't impact her all that much. Chrissy had a bodacious body that made teenage boys crazy, big brown eyes that didn't miss a trick and a mind made for navigating the social shoals of adolescence. Like me, she had done some hard time at private school for many of the same reasons, planned a dramatic escape and was happily ensconced in (hold your breath) the public high school.

We were lying out in the sun in the backyard of Chrissy's parents' split-level ranch, draped out across heavy, metal trifold chairs with the thick plastic strapping that made creases in your face if you fell asleep on your stomach. Basking in the sun in my one-piece bathing suit, staring into space, listening to Chrissy sing every lyric to every song that played on the Top 40 radio station and roasting my skin with baby oil made me happy that day.

For a little bit, I fit in somewhere. With my friend, mind you, who had social currency to spare and generously decided to spend some on me.

While there were many great things about Chrissy, one of her fabulous traits was her keen interest in the details and minutiae of your life. The other was her uncanny ability to recall all of those details and minutiae of your life. I mean it, she remembered it all, down to the last detail of how you wore your hair and what you were wearing, as well as how she wore *her* hair and what *she* was wearing, when you told her the details and minutiae of your life.

That afternoon, laid out prone, I recounted my tale of social woe. She listened with vigilance. She asked succinct questions at the right moments. She pondered and contemplated and finally sprang up on her elbows, holding her untied bikini up against her very well-endowed chest.

"Well, after all that crap, you'll just have to find a date," she announced. She said it so simply that she made it sound possible. And for her, it was. But for me, it was like scaling Mount Everest: I didn't have the skills, the stamina or the training to take on such a Herculean task without losing some fingers or toes—or my life. I told her as much.

"Don't be silly," she shot back as she strategically positioned her bathing-suit top and adjusted her sunglasses. "Why don't you ask Hunter?"

Hunter was Chrissy's younger brother. As such, he was like my brother. I had known him since preschool; we likely had peed together in the pool on family vacation. In fact, he was such a part of my family landscape that he barely registered on my radar, beyond me snickering at how his southern mama said his name: "Hun-tuh."

The fact that Hun-tuh didn't register on my radar was unusual, because he was tall, rowdy, fun, very funny and, according to some, good-looking. A blond version of Chrissy—shiny white teeth and all.

"Going with Hunter is like going with my brother," I said. It felt weird and a bit alien to me.

"Who cares?" Chrissy countered. "He'll be a great date and you'll have a fun time—which is more than anyone can say for that Raymond dude." She wrinkled her nose in distaste on my behalf and turned away to change the station on the radio. She was right. Hunter would be a great date, and I would have a fun time.

Later that afternoon, Hunter loped through the yard on his way home from a friend's house and Chrissy yelled, "Hey, Hunter, hold up for a second! Charla wants to ask you something."

Now, you might think that could have been an awkward setup, or that I was about to have an awkward moment. But this was Hunter, my annoying but clever pseudo little brother. He walked over.

"I have this dance to go to in a few weeks and I need a date. Do you want to go?"

He paused. "Who else will be there?" Again, you might construe this as an awkward or even rude question. But this was Hunter, my annoying but clever, and very confident, pseudo little brother.

"It will be fun. A lot of those cute girls who are friends with Amy and Julie will be there—it's their prom." He processed that little socially enticing tidbit. "Sure. Okay. Sounds fun." And he walked into the house to watch television, and that was that. Chrissy threw a reassuring smile my way, settled down into her sun-goddess position and got ready for the next round. "Now, what are you going to wear?"

Showing up with Hunter as my date to my ninth-grade prom at a school where I struggled to outrun my reputation as the cross-dressing interloper who played woodwinds was one of Chrissy's more fabulous plans. I wore a simple sundress with spaghetti straps, a fitted bodice and a skirt with box pleats. It was dotted with azure-blue flowers the size of golf balls and topped with a cardigan sweater. And I did have fun. And I did dance. And I wouldn't have to pine for a kiss or outmaneuver one. What I didn't count on was the impact that my date would have on the entire evening.

Hunter showed up in a light blue three-piece suit—a comic contrast to the other boys' khaki pants and navy blazers. With his ersatz-cool vibe, he danced and talked and charmed. It was as if I had taken the Justin Timberlake of Asheville, North Carolina, to the prom. People were equal parts impressed, surprised and suspicious. They eyed him cautiously, not sure what to do with him.

During a dance, Hunter gave me a wink and a grin—as if he and I were the ones on the inside of some big joke. The wink that said, "I can't believe how easy this is, can you?" A grin that said, "You know you can't take any of this seriously, right?"

As I looked around that small gym, festooned with aluminum-foil decor and a handmade vignette that featured a shaky staircase making a lopsided reach toward heaven, my focus shifted. My world, which for the last nine months had been small and narrow, defined by a small and narrow group of people (including the likes of Raymond Reynolds, the Johnson twins and me), suddenly relaxed. I realized that this version of reality—the one where I played the awkward new girl who didn't quite fit in, didn't make the cut for the girls' basketball team and didn't get asked to the ninth-grade prom—didn't have to be my reality forever.

I recognized that starting tomorrow, I could sail away from this reality and find a different group of people who didn't remember me as the awkwardly garbed gal with the phallic flute. And this isn't just true of middle school—this is true every day, in the real world, no matter what your age. That's what I love about it—so many chances to meet new people and make a new first impression, or, impress upon them that you're not always going to be the same girl that they used to know.

And as the years go by, we become a bit more practiced about how to present ourselves. For example, in my Pretty City, we pride ourselves on making a good first impression, and that includes making people feel welcome, whether it be in our homes or to the neighborhood. A family just moved from California to a prestigious neighborhood in my hometown. The husband is a fabulously successful entrepreneur. The wife is a California beauty. They have two lovely children, who were immediately accepted and enrolled in one of the top private schools in the city. They bought an incredibly fabulous house, and since their arrival, they have been feted at no less than a dozen social events—coffees, cocktails and dinner parties. All in their honor—to welcome them to town, to introduce them, to connect them. Their dance card was filled so quickly, in fact, that it was rumored that the wife had to start *declining* offers from hospitable folks who wanted to meet, greet and introduce them to the who's who of our fair southern city.

My friend Aimee, when hearing all of this straight from the horse's mouth (as she was invited to one of these meet-and-greet soirees) astutely noted to me at Book Club one evening, "All I got when I moved to town was a loaf of banana bread and a neighborhood directory."

As it turns out, this couple was so dazzling and shiny, and hailed from the Prettiest State in the Union, that their first impression preceded them. We should all be so lucky. Likewise, my Pretty City was eager to make a good first impression, too. I wondered what this couple made of their new city and new friends. Did they enjoy them? Were they cloying? Did their hands cramp from writing all those thank-you notes?

It may seem antiquated or trivial or downright silly to worry about things like a well-written thank-you note, or the proper funeral suit, or the ideal casserole to deliver to the new neighbor who just had a baby. But right or wrong, all these niceties (or expectations, depending on your point of view) are a way of life—or at least the life I know.

For those of us steeped in southern culture like tea bags steeping in the sun, it's a life that feels comfortable and good. In the space between *Gone With the Wind* and *My Big Fat Redneck Wedding* lives a large portion of the rest of us, working diligently to show the world that our parents *raised us right*. After all, first impressions are a way of maintaining civility and order in our world and often that's not all bad. But what's interesting is when others don't share your first-impression priority.

There's a wonderful hairdresser in town who my friend Tracey goes to. Jannie is a true southern woman from the tips of her stylish blond hair to her bronze sandals. She could easily star in her own version of *Steel Magnolias* (minus the cemetery scene) as she rattles off bits of wisdom and bons mots just as fast as Dolly Parton can slip on a wig. Jannie knows exactly what she likes and, after a trip to New York City to attend a hair convention, knows that she DOES. NOT. LIKE. NEW. YORK. CITY. "For Pete's sake, I have never had so many doors closed on me in my entire life. Does no one in the North hold the door for a woman? I was about to cry!" Jannie exclaimed. But worse than aching feet, slammed doors and rude cabbies was the sad observation that, according to Jannie's strong southern sensibility, so few women cared about how they looked.

"I sat in a Starbucks and I saw one woman after the other

coming up out of the subway in some hideous shapeless coat that made these girls look like overgrown Oompa-Loompas. And here's the worst—wet hair and no makeup. Can you believe it? Going out in public like that? Who goes outside with wet hair besides seniors leaving their water-aerobics class? I wanted to do an intervention, just stand out there with a tube of lip gloss and say to them, 'Stand still, let me put this on you. It will *change* your *life.*'"

How did Jannie know this? How did she know that lip gloss and a spot of mascara could change one's life? Because Jannie knew the fundamental truth of first impressions—at their core, they make a difference, if only to the person making them. And at the very least, that counts for something.

When folks who had never met me discovered I was writing a book about daily intimacy with my spouse (not the mailman, not my personal trainer, not my dentist . . . but my *husband*), it altered the first impression I made. It also altered others' impression of those who had known me for years. Even my parents.

When I delicately shared with my mother that I had an offer to publish a book, she squealed, "I just knew you would write a children's book one day!" But when the sober reality set in that I would be writing a memoir (i.e., a *true story* about life behind closed bedroom doors), it was a bit of a shock.

"What are you going to tell your father?" she asked me.

"I was hoping you would tell him," I replied, perpetuating a long-standing tradition of passive familial communications.

My mother, never one to shirk the opportunity to insert her-self in the thick of family drama, rallied. "I'll try," she said.

Finally, my father called me one afternoon.

"Are you getting paid to write this book?" asked my dad as we sorted through the details of this extraordinarily whacked-out idea of a nice southern girl like me writing a book about you-know-what.

"Of course I'm getting paid to write this book," I answered. "By a very reputable publishing house in New York City. They're giving me an advance."

"I see," he said. "Well, whatever they're paying you to publish it, I'll pay you double NOT to publish it."

Like it or not, my family was going to be deeply impacted by my decision to publish a memoir about marriage and intimacy. And they were worried (rightfully so) that I was underestimating how deeply impacted I could be by my decision to publish a memoir about my marriage and the role intimacy played in it. What I realized only later, when it was far too late to contemplate, second-guess or turn back time, was that in many ways, that book, my decision, this very public declaration, would forever become part of my first impression. Like the fabulous couple whose reputation and first impression preceded their move to my Pretty City, my first impression would precede me, too.

Fast-forward to a dinner I was having with a group of women who had invited me to serve alongside them on a yearlong vol-unteer committee. As we wrapped up dinner, someone casually mentioned my *Oprah* appearance. The other women sat up and took note and I cautiously absorbed their reactions as they slowly realized that I was the one who wrote THAT BOOK.

One woman choked on her Pinot Noir, and her big brown eyes grew wide. Another was rendered speechless and looked around for confirmation of the same. After an awkward, pregnant pause, peals of laughter erupted and the questions started flying. Later, after the usual dishing about talk-show hosts and bad reviews, one of the women, Kiki, turned to me.

"We've been working together on this committee for nearly six months! How in the world did we not know you wrote that book?" she asked.

"Sometimes it works out better when people know me first. Especially a group of fabulously committed women who open every meeting with prayer," I added with a wry smile.

What I had discovered AFTER the book publicity tour, and what I shared with Kiki, was that the book didn't have to define me. I'm so much more than what people read (and choose to write) about me. Most people are. I discovered that when people get to know me first, the book becomes an interesting and organic part of the conversation when the time is right and not a titillating headline that can cast an impression that often isn't accurate. Please know that I just didn't wake up one day so emotionally healthy and well balanced. It took me a good eighteen months to arrive at this Zen-like state.

Kiki tilted her head, took a lingering sip of her Pinot and paused. "I think you're right," she said. "I think it's fabulous you wrote that book. And the reason I think it's fabulous is because

I know YOU." She did know me—she knew my sense of commitment, my sense of humor, my strange sense of modesty and more.

And then she grinned and added, "I am so having you over for dinner. My husband is not going to believe this. It's going to be great!" And she did and he didn't and it was.

One of the many lessons learned from this book experience was the idea that I might order people's impressions of me. It didn't always work, of course. Because at the end of the day, there are some first impressions you can control and there are some you can't. Some people will love you because of who you are or what you did or what you can do for them. And some people will never be able to shake that first impression of you— the one from the first day at a new school or the night you were severely overserved at an outdoor concert or the time you wore those really cheap, plastic shoes to work. It's not right and it's not fair, it just is. That's why first impressions really are important—not because they can smack of false airs and pretenses and affectations. Rather, first impressions count because they are a powerful, one-of-a-kind opportunity to serve up your best self. *E Pluribus Unum*, I say.

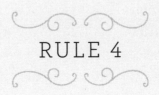

RULE 4

Own It

Everyone called him Oscar, as though they had been friends for years and hadn't just been introduced.

He was taller than I imagined. Not over six feet, but taller than some of the oh-so-petite famous folks. And tan. It was a deep, dark tan, likely manufactured, but it suited him. He was dashing and trim in a well-cut suit and had this fabulously thick Latin accent. And yes, he was sexy, even at almost eighty years old. If you think a married man this age can't be sexy, attractive and totally and thoroughly modern, then you've never met Oscar de la Renta.

First, let's get a few things straight.

Meeting one of the world's preeminent fashion designers was not going to bring anyone one step closer to world peace, close the deficit gap, or better educate America's children. And meeting him would not change the core of who I was, nor would it make me a better person. But this was the man who said, "I have always felt my role as a designer is to do the very best I can for a woman to make her look her best." "Hallelujah" is all I can say. I need all the help I can get. Needless to say, I fell for him long before I set eyes on him in May 2011 and would spend several months leading up to that month preparing to meet him.

In my Pretty City, May is one of the high holy months of Pretty and the perfect time for Oscar to visit. The azaleas are in full bloom and our famously tree-lined streets grow shaded with a heavy canopy of lush green leaves. Charlotte's major museum hosts a series of fund-raisers each spring—home tours, garden parties, black-tie galas and symposiums featuring fancy New York City interior designers with names like Bunny and Miles. It's a week of pretty—gorgeous two-piece silk-blend suits the color of hydrangeas; beautiful baubles carefully unpacked from the safe; marvelously manicured feet tucked into mile-high Manolos, pretty Carmen Marc Valvo sheath dresses and impeccably styled tresses with just the right amount of sun-kissed highlights. For the Ladies Who Lunch (and Donate) set, it's a monthlong frenzy of preparation, shopping, tailoring and showing up ready to present their look to their fellow (hopefully) admiring crowd.

This particular year's event was special—one of the organizers grew up with Oscar de la Renta's lovely stepdaughter and she helped tee up a special event that would feature Oscar de la Renta, a "real" runway show with "real" runway models strutting his fall collection, and a glittering collection of our city's finest in their finest—all to raise money for our art museum, which boasts a rather impressive costume and dress collection.

And I was invited to do the PR for the event. I know! Pinch me.

It was an incredible opportunity that doesn't come along often if, say, you live ANYWHERE outside New York City, Milan or Paris. So I juggled and rearranged and created enough time in my schedule to accept this grand job offer.

"I'm in," I told the Pretty Girls in Charge, who worked tirelessly for the better part of a year before I entered stage left. I sat in meeting after meeting with gals who gave a new definition to the words "high achiever." These were smart, connected and impeccably well-dressed women with beautiful hair. To boot, they were a pleasure to work with. They welcomed new ideas, they got things done, they asked nicely and they looked great doing it.

It would have been so easy to hate them. I tried for a minute or two, but it didn't work.

Instead, I focused on what to wear at each gathering, as every planning meeting, committee regroup, reception and lunch became a study in personal grooming. I was running out of clothes to wear and the actual events were more than a month away. My iron and my alterationist, Marine Sergeant Marie, had not seen this kind of action or so much of me since—well, ever. But still, this was a once-in-a-lifetime gig, and I could make my sweater sets last at least that long.

In one meeting, about six months out, the Pretty Girls casually discussed what to wear to each event: the gala, the symposium, the luncheon, the backyard band party. "Well, I think it's appropriate—and somewhat expected—that some of us will wear Oscar to the gala," said one, she-who-stands-nearly-six-feet-tall-in-bare-feet. My ears twitched.

"I know, I've been in touch with some of my favorite shops in L.A. about some possibilities," said another, a gorgeous Raphaelite blonde who owns one of the city's most chic boutiques and has skin so luminous I swear she must shimmer in her sleep. They continued to compare notes on Oscar gowns, and I started to pit out. It's a good thing I was wearing a cardigan.

Donning an Oscar de la Renta gown at an Oscar de la Renta event where Oscar de la Renta would be the guest of honor reeks of common sense and good graces. But I couldn't afford to buy an Oscar and certainly don't qualify to rent couture gowns: they can't be altered. At five foot three inches (on a good day), everything I own, rent or shoplift (not really) must be hemmed.

I felt a bit out of sorts, sitting between these fashion-forward gals whom I ventured never ran errands in smelly gym clothes or with their hair bobby-pinned out of the way. There I was: a regular Jane both in pocketbook and height, uncertain of how I'd make do.

So a few months prior to the big event, when one of our city's most chic boutiques hosted a champagne reception where they displayed racks and racks of gorgeous Oscar de la Renta frocks, I did a pop-in to check things out. Fashion-forward gals were gliding around the sunlit boutique, gliding into luxe dressing rooms to don dresses. Thirty- and forty-something Cinderellas picking out an Oscar for the ball. It's true—everyone looks lovely in an Oscar. I cautiously thumbed through the racks, making sure my hands were impeccably clean. Who wants to be the schmuck who smudges an Oscar? The fabrics were exquisite, the construction impeccable, the designs dreamlike. I stuffed back panic. Meeting Oscar de la Renta is one thing. Financing him is quite another. I was out of my couture league—as if any couture was ever in my league.

So instead, to make myself feel more at home, I went to a women's retail store that I often frequent. Granted, it's fairly conservative, but the price point fits my wallet. Not to mention, they have a great petites section and killer sales. Before making my way to the formal wear, I spotted a rack of cardigans in every imaginable color. Naturally, I stopped to thumb through the rack. It's no secret that I am a cardigan fanatic—I am obsessed with them. I have at least two dozen cardigans in a rainbow of colors and shades. Mostly a cotton-Lycra blend (for just enough stretch and fit), but a few in lovely cashmere, and one in angora wool (holy moly, does it shed). I have scoop neck, V-neck and some come with sweet pearl buttons. One has rhinestone buttons for some cardigan pizzazz! Cardis are the ultimate in versatility and work great down south—there is NOTHING that doesn't go with a good cardigan, and in my Pretty City, you can wear them all year round. A cardigan can be spiffed up, down and sideways. I keep my cardigans carefully folded in a wide dresser, arranged in Roy G. Biv fashion. It's like a secret rainbow tucked in my drawer, guaranteed to bring a smile even on the dreariest of days.

I was shopping at said store, which was having a killer sale, sorting through my dream rack, when a woman approached me and started doing the same. She was petite, older than I but younger than my mother. I turned to her to share my enthusiasm.

"Don't you just love these sweaters? The colors are always so pretty and the weight is perfect—they're nearly all-season." I attempted to create some cardi-solidarity.

"I know," agreed the woman. "They're terrific. I buy them in every color. For my mother. She's eighty-nine and lives at the Methodist Home, and she's always complaining that her room is cold. She just loves these cardigans."

I froze.

Time stopped. Sound and color dropped away and all I could hear was this: "My mother loves these cardigans . . . she's eighty-nine . . . my mother loves these cardigans . . . she's eighty-nine . . ."

I stood with a stack of four sweaters and stared catatonically into space, visions of octogenarians sitting in the TV room at the Methodist Home watching *The Price Is Right*, each with a different-colored cardi draped around her hunched shoulders. My cardis, the ones that "go" with everything, apparently go well with Bob Barker and Depends.

Carefully laying all the cardigans back on the sales shelf, I turned wordlessly and left the store. Apparently my personal style mantra was one cardigan away from staid old ladies who put their teeth in for lunch.

There I was, with the incredible fashion burden of dressing

for an Oscar de la Renta event on a Target budget and with an octogenarian's fashion sense.

I was so hosed.

I've known that I've always had a bent for the conservative, but who knew it was a conservative that had tipped dangerously close to the doddering. And I'll fess up to once owning a dog-eared copy of *The Preppy Handbook*. I think all women look great in a classic wrap dress, sling-back pumps and some well-placed bling (real or faux). A man in white bucks and a bow tie makes me weak in the knees. That doesn't mean that I don't like and appreciate the Sultry Siren or Boho Chic look of some of my friends, it's just that I know I can't pull it off.

I find it hard enough to present well within the context of Traditional Preppy with a Southern Twist, so asking me to be some sort of Pucci Princess or Bohemian Babe? Not gonna happen.

When I am asked by my friends or family for fashion input, it's not surprising I can be mildly reliable only if someone is dressing in my fashion wheelhouse. You want feedback on tailored suits, classic Tod flats and pashmina wraps? I'm your girl.

Case in point, my dear friend Kate attended a late-summer wedding in the mountains. She shopped all over Pretty City for the right dress, finally settling on a gorgeous Kay Unger garment from Neiman's. It was beautiful—a satin bodice and tweedy bouclé skirt. It was a gentle slate-blue color and sleeveless. She hemmed it just above the knee. Kate has thin, shapely calves and ankles and found a pair of strappy sandals in a pearly gray. She paired it with a pretty pashmina and a sassy clutch purse (both courtesy of *moi*).

That fall, she lamented the fact that she had nothing to wear to one of THE Christmas parties of the season (which she hosts along with me and our friend Caroline). Of course, I thought the gentle slate-blue Kay Unger dress would be perfect. It was the epitome of transitional, after all.

"I don't know, Char, I know the dress is pretty and all," said Kate. "But it just seems matronly."

Matronly? I LOVED this dress—it was sleeveless, short and formfitting, not some Mama Cass caftan (and it's not like she was wearing a cardigan with it). Admittedly it was traditional, nonedgy and "very appropriate," as my mother would say. But that's what made it perfect for a holiday cocktail party, or so I thought.

Instead, Kate wore black Kate Spade booties, black jeggings and a killer sweater dress laced with silver thread and all sorts of cool jangle jewelry. Kind of Joan Jett meets Trendy Gallery Owner. She looked great, of course. Me? I went another route and opted for a vintage debut.

I decided to wear an LBD that had belonged to my father's sister some sixty years ago. Made of black crepe, it had a sheer black overlay for the sleeves and back. A dainty belt the width of a ruler with two little black snaps to hold it in place. It was retro chic and remarkably intact, considering its age. My mother discovered it in the back of a cedar-lined storage closet in the basement of her house, dusted if off and passed it my way.

At first, I didn't think I could make it work—even after having lost weight. It was so small, I wasn't sure I could pull it up over my hips and I certainly couldn't wear a bra, as it barely fit across my rib cage. My mom gingerly manhandled the side zipper, catching a big chunk of my skin in the process. But then the zipper zipped, and the dress fit. She and I both looked in the mirror.

The fact that this dress fit me was secondary to *how* this dress fit me—it was haunting, like a fashion poltergeist. As my mother had pointed out to me at a ripe young age, I am high-waisted, but this dress gathered and draped at my thinnest part. I am short, but this dress hit me at the sweet spot—the upper third of my kneecap. There was a hidden lace trim across the neckline that we discovered and carefully unfolded and re-shaped. It softened the broadness of my shoulders. It was as if someone had made this dress for me. Which of course they hadn't, because someone made it for my aunt Henrietta, who was born in 1921 and likely wore it during her courtship.

We looked for a label but there was nothing—not one clue sewn into the dress to give us a hint of its lineage. We asked my father and he gave some vague response about his mother commissioning dresses to be designed and sewn for his two older sisters. He saw me in his sister's dress, and I couldn't interpret the memories that flashed across his face. While I look nothing like my father or his family, the fit of this dress was uncanny. It was a sign, I thought. Of what? I had no idea.

I decided to wear the dress to the holiday party. It would be a stark contrast to the two other hostesses—Kate's fashion-forward, of-the-moment holiday attire and Caroline's glittery

silver strappy frock and stiletto shoes. But I adored the dress—
loved that it had a story that didn't belong to me. Also, I loved
that this dress might collect some new stories, too. But mostly, I
loved that I could zip up the freakin' thing.

Of course, an hour before the party I panicked.

"What was I thinking!" I lamented to Brad as I pulled on my
special occasion, industrial-strength Spanx. "I can't wear this
used, washed-up dress that's been hanging in a cedar closet for
sixty years—I will look ridiculous, ancient! Does it smell? I swear
I think it still smells fusty. Here, smell my thigh." I kicked up my
leg for a sniff test and apparently passed. At the very least I can
count on Brad to tell me if I reek.

"You're going to look great," he said. He donned his White
Man Uniform—flat-front gabardine trousers, Brooks Brothers
dress shirt and cashmere V-neck sweater—and went to watch
SportsCenter while I teetered on the brink of a fashion melt-
down. This time as Clara Bow Flapper Gone Bad. But it was too
late, I didn't have time. In less than an hour, more than three
hundred people would show up for this party and I would be
there to meet, greet and air-kiss the night away in a flimsy un-
lined crepe dress that smelled like mothballs. Move over, Queen
Mother, there is a new dowdy in Pretty City . . . and it's yours
truly!

As I started to pace around my room fiddling with my jewelry, I realized there was nothing I could do. I had no backup
outfit for this night, no Plan B that included fashion from this
decade. So I straightened my shoulders. Gave my hair an extra
few shots of hair spray. Applied another layer of my Chanel Lip

Glossimer. Grabbed my pashmina and sling-back pumps and headed out the door.

Of course, the party was terrific. The food was delicious, the decor was twinkly and bright and the guests just as sparkly. When one is circulating among three hundred of your closest friends in a happy champagne haze, no one seems to notice one's unpedigreed, slightly odiferous LBD. Instead, I received some very lovely compliments and regaled a guest or two with the story of its mysterious origins. Despite my mini fashion melt-down, it really was my kind of dress—classic lines, a simple design and an interesting story. While it would be easy to say I got lucky that evening with my LBD, what transpired was actually a little glimpse into some personal fashion growth. An experience in what not only looks good but, more important, feels good on me. It only took forty-something years, but it was a valuable lesson.

And while that dress saved me on more than one occasion, I still had an Oscar problem to contend with and needed a fashion intervention from a higher power. And since "couture" and "affordable" go together about as well as white patent leather shoes and winter, I knew I had to be creative. More creative than I had been when I hired an image consultant before hopping on the Talk Show Train to Hell. How I didn't realize that dressing to "blend in" when you're on national television talking about your sex life is a paradox of epic proportions still stumps me. And to this day, my mother stands by her claim that less than half of my guided purchases were "wearable," whatever the heck that means. Since we had the same coloring, the same build and roughly the same hairstyle, what looked good on her nearly always looked good on me, and so she shared her opinions freely. What I think she was really trying to hint at was that I was looking a fashion gift horse in the mouth, so to speak, and had no need to waste hard-earned money on a fashion consultant.

I thought about asking my mother for advice this time around, but instead I surfed eBay for hours upon hours upon hours. I found other websites, too—consignment stores in Dallas, Los Angeles, New York and Chicago. Yes, there are vintage Oscar dresses to be had. But how do you close the deal on a dress that costs nearly as much as your wedding gown but has a no-return policy? What if it doesn't fit? What if the color isn't right? What if your tiny little chest doesn't fill out the dress? And we all know that a size twelve in a couture dress is like a size four in off-the-rack dresses (at least I knew this, after burning dozens of hours checking out dresses). I simply couldn't pull the online trigger. I fretted and did absolutely nothing. But then again, there wasn't some Oscar dream dress out there in cyberspace that I just had to have, a dress that was so beautiful, so "Charla" and so dead-on appropriate for my Oscar gala that I couldn't live without it.

I floated along like a man without a country—okay, I was just a girl without a dress. I continued to attend the gala planning meetings where the women discreetly chatted about which Oscar they were wearing to which event, about shopping trips to Atlanta and New York City, about accessories and shoes and jewelry. I just continued to pop Tums, wipe my sweaty palms on my wool pants and say nothing.

Then one morning in February, while I was lying in bed in my parents' house in Florida, an idea finally struck me. My kids and I were spending a long weekend enjoying the sunny skies of the Sunshine State. I sat bolt upright and silently applauded myself. For the love of couture, my snowbird parents live in Palm Beach County—home to things high end, expensive, formal and worn only once! I jumped out of bed, hopped onto the laptop and Googled *consignment shops, Palm Beach.* The flood of names that popped on my screen made me swoon with joy. I had hit a mother lode, and my mother could go with me to load up.

Please, please, please, I thought to myself as I spiffed up for a spontaneous trek to Palm Beach, *let me find an Oscar de la Renta on deep, deep,* deep *discount.*

The consignment and vintage shops in Palm Beach are nestled together in a five-block radius right off Worth Avenue. No matter the high-end real estate, they still have the cheesiest names, like Attitudes and Razamataz. I mean, really? But Classic Closet seemed okay. It was dark and crowded and a Glamour Shot of the owner, Mary, hung over the cash register. My mother was buzzing around the store manager—a woman on an Oscar mission. I have to say this about my mother: if you give her a very specific task, very specific details and a very specific time frame, the woman is on fire. And if that task involves shopping and keeping sales associates on their toes? Then all I can tell you is to get out of the way.

"My daughter is attending a gala in Charlotte for Oscar de la Renta where Mr. de la Renta will be in attendance," she said. "We are only interested in Oscar dresses that are appropriate to spring in a mild climate." The woman started sorting through the racks and pulling out options. There were too many Oscar dresses to be believed.

"Black velvet in April? No thank you," my mother commented to one with a wave of her hand. "Chartreuse is not her color," she said to another. "That is much too small," she offered with a nod. Shopgirls paraded through, nodding respectfully to my mother as she sent them away.

Then a full-length sheath the color of Chanel lipstick No. 5 appeared, dramatically draped over the arm of an older sales associate. My mom and I locked gazes and our eyes twinkled. We are both red girls and this dress was the perfect red—not an orangey tomato red, but a deep, blue-based red the color of ripe cherries. The color that makes our olive complexions and dark hair and eyes pop. It was satin with an incredible hand-sewn bustier that forced a posture I had never known existed in my spine. And down the back was the most soft, graceful draping that I had ever seen, like a beautiful red waterfall.

My mother crammed into the too-tiny dressing room to help me wedge into the dress. There were hooks and drawstrings and two different zippers to maneuver the fabric around me. The fit of the dress pulled back my shoulders and tilted my chin upward, forcing me into a sort of regal stance that only royalty are forced to perfect.

I walked out of the dressing room to the three-way mirror. Mary and the shopgirls clustered around me like hens.

"Oh my gawd, that dress was made for you!"

"That color is incredible!"

"It doesn't need to be hemmed or altered, it's a perfect fit."

"It's the most gorgeous dress . . . you have to get it."

And then Mary, the consummate professional, stepped into center stage with me and cast her discerning gaze my way. She pulled and prodded, checking the fit and making adjustments. She nodded and agreed. "This dress looks incredible on you. You have to get it. I'll check, but I think I can give you fifteen percent off the current price."

My mother and I hadn't even glanced at the tag on the red dress. I wasn't ready. I felt like Eliza Doolittle, but in a dark, secondhand shop in Florida, and I wanted to have my little fairy-tale moment a minute longer. Bathed in bad light in front of a three-way mirror, I simply absorbed the red dress. The way it fit my body and hugged my curves and nudged my posture. For that short moment in time, I felt amazing. When you're in your early forties, you gotta grab 'em when you can.

Then my mother looked at the price tag, made a choking sound and rocked around the store until she found a stool to collapse on. So much for my moment. Then I looked, too, made a choking sound and joined her. Ugh, I could never pay that much money for a dress. Even a dress *that* transforming.

Mary was buzzing around, trying to be helpful, talking about payment plans and layaway and all sorts of nonsense. My mom and I exchanged a few comments while I threw on my clothes.

"Honey, it's gorgeous, it fits you like a glove. It's a forever dress—but the price tag . . ."

"Mom, I know. It's just too much. But isn't it the most beautiful thing you've ever seen?"

"Yes, and you look beautiful in it, honey, you really do. Let's visit some other stores and think about it."

"I can't think about it. Brad would divorce me if I bought a dress that expensive."

We went back and forth and back and forth as we exited the store and hit the other shops for a look-see. But it was a half-hearted effort, we both knew. THE DRESS was hanging back in Mary's shop, waiting for me.

All told, it was an incredibly fun day—I had never actually gone shopping for couture gowns before, and trying them on, albeit at a series of first-rate secondhand stores, was a whole new experience. Kind of like discovering that chateaubriand is indeed way better than a burger. But I was a bit melancholy, too, back to square one on my quest to find a dress.

Later that evening, my mom came to my room. She stood in the doorway, her hand on the knob, eyes soft with affection. "If you ever tell Brad I did this, I will deny it and then kill you later. But let's figure out a way to get the dress."

I should tell you that I was stunned by the offer, I really was. But in many ways, I wasn't.

Not because I am some presumptuous forty-something brat who expects her parents to buy her stuff, but rather because my mother has an incredibly generous and gentle streak in her, despite her efficient nature. She's sneaky that way. She saw and understood what I felt that day. And like many mothers, she wanted to help make it happen. She wanted me to look great and feel great. But that didn't mean I was going to let her. After all, I was an adult and I did have a little something called pride.

Besides, my husband would kill me if he knew *anyone* paid that much for a dress. So we battled back and forth and back and forth. Then the next morning I called Mary.

(You knew I would, didn't you?)

"Mary," I told her, wearing my most serious negotiating face, which she couldn't appreciate by phone. "I really want that dress. But I have two conditions," I said, and I meant it. "What is the absolute best you can do on the cost? And you must tell me who owned this dress."

The first condition was de rigueur, the second one was a real no-no. And I knew it. It was gauche and inappropriate to tattle about which socialites were moving their frocks and gowns through consignment shops. While some were merely unloading gowns they had worn once or twice to make room for new ones, others were making discreet deliveries to the back doors of the shops because they were short on cash and long on couture. Mary's clientele counted on her discretion for all kinds of reasons. It didn't matter; I still wanted to know. It was the voyeur in me. Who was this women who wore the simple red Oscar gown? Where did she wear it? How did she feel in it? If I could get a detail or two of her story, I could spin out the tale and layer her story into mine.

After I did a double-pinky swear and gave her my shipping information and the credit card, Mary told me. I grinned in delight. It was such a tantalizing little piece of information that made the Oscar dress—now MY Oscar dress—that much more wonderful. Much like an antique sideboard or your grandmother's silver pitcher, the dress had a story. A story I would continue.

Before you get all "Circle of Life" on me and start mocking my nostalgia, let me say this: I was set with a killer Oscar dress for my killer Oscar event featuring Oscar de la Renta himself.

Or so I thought.

I returned from Florida and was sitting in another Oscar planning meeting. The beautiful boutique owner with the china-doll skin was chatting with the six-foot glamazon about the dress code for the event. One was thinking about cocktail pants. The other had her eye on a vintage jacket.

"Wait a minute," I interrupted. "You mean this event is not black tie?"

"Nope," one responded. "We decided to make it 'From Casual to Couture' in order to invite people to be fashionably creative and comfortable. We don't want the event to look like prom night."

Really, I should use prescription deodorant. My face turned red, my breath shortened and my head started to spin. I had just shopped all over freakin' Kingdom Come, purchased (and set up a payment plan for my mother) a formal Oscar de la Renta gown to wear to the event of the year and I'm going to be *overdressed*? I'm going to be mingling with men in sport coats and women in couture work attire?

Kill me now and steal my jewelry, why don't you?

These were nice girls and they started clucking over my slight panic attack. I confessed to my recent couture purchase. "Don't worry, wear the dress. You'll look fine," one said. Fine? I wanted to scream. For that amount of dough and angst and stress, I needed to look *way* more than fine, I thought. I needed to look divinely appropriate and totally fabulous.

"Listen, I'll help you accessorize," the other said. "Just don't wear pearls or rhinestones, you know? You can dress it down with a cool cuff and gladiator sandals or something"

I nearly choked. Pairing the only couture gown I would ever own with a cuff and Jesus footwear? Things had just gone from bad to worse.

I couldn't even scream and cry about it—there was no one I could let in on my pathetic little fashion debacle. My husband would kill me. My mother would be crushed. My painfully pragmatic and sensible friend Cyndee would tell me I was an idiot in the first place. And she'd be right.

I was so angry I could hardly look at myself in the mirror. For three days, I walked around in a state of emotional self-flagellation. Cursing myself. Cursing my mother's über-generosity. Cursing my naivete. And on the fourth day, I snapped out of it.

Listen, I told myself one day, while peering into my triple-magnifying mirror to do some serious plucking and tweezing. *It's done,* I told my giant nostril. *You own the dress. You can't return it. Your mother did something incredibly lovely and generous to help you. The dress looks great on you. It's going to be an amazing evening. You can make it work. What you need to do now is OWN IT.*

Own it. Own it. Own it.

And I didn't just tell myself to own the dress. I needed to own the experience. Own my part in making it happen. Own my right to wear that dress and look flip-out fabulous, even if it durn near killed me.

So I did.

I met Oscar, I sat in his suite at the Ritz-Carlton and I listened to him tell stories in his Dominican accent. He was charming and handsome and current and I tried mightily to commit every second of it to memory. I wore an incredibly beautiful and bold red gown that I discovered while shopping with a fab mom. I wore a simple pair of earrings and my wedding band. I had a great blowout and sported luscious fake eyelashes. I watched a swank, big-city fashion show live and up close, and I drank champagne from a sparkly fluted glass. I paused while two women oohed and aahed and took a picture of the red waterfall down the back of my dress. Some people didn't recognize me. Others pretended not to be surprised when they ran into me. Either way, I didn't care.

This was my Oscar night and I owned it.

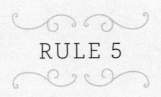

RULE 5

Be at Peace with
What You're Not

I was in the fourth grade when I realized that Kelly Pringle had the most amazing, knock-your-socks-off dimples. She had one perfectly placed movie-star dimple on each cheek that rendered her face impossibly beautiful. Dimples so deep and pronounced that I could probably wedge a dime in one and it would stay put. Who needed a round, heart-shaped face with a slight double chin when you could have showstopping dimples just like Kelly Pringle?

Dimples, I just knew, would change my life. I *needed* dimples. I would be prettier and more popular and make better grades. And since I was a fairly industrious ten-year-old, I decided I would get me some.

So one afternoon, I started rummaging through my mother's jewelry drawer—yes, it was a very big drawer. Back in the seventies, I would venture to say that no one had just one jewelry box. A box simply could not hold all of that funky, groovy, dangly, psychedelic costume jewelry that was so in style. In that oversize trove of costume treasures, I found an inexpensive choker with a ball-and-hook clasp. It was a stiff choker, and when I pulled it open, it reverbed with just enough tension. My wheels got to turning.

Standing in front of the mirror, I carefully wedged one end of the choker in one cheek and the other end of the necklace in the other. It wasn't uncomfortable, but it was stiff enough that it stuck—providing enough rigid pressure, or so I thought, to create in each cheek the beautiful divot that I coveted. Imagine orthodontic headgear . . . but wedged at a slightly different angle. No pain, no gain, I figured as I strutted to my room donning a jerry-rigged facial apparatus that would make any anesthetist proud. Good-bye, pudgy, heart-shaped cheeks. Hello, knee-deep dimples.

Of course, my first stint at noninvasive plastic surgery failed. But thus was born my lifelong quest to change, tweak or otherwise alter what the good Lord gave me.

I know that we are all wonderfully and purposefully made—my church and my parents taught me this from an early age. But on many days, I have drunk the punch of pop culture and am acting president of the SPAM Club (Society of Please Accept Me). It is hard to not become preoccupied with wrinkles, cellulite and keratin treatments. That's when I'm consumed by the urge to fix, change, alter, adjust and will away the exact elements I'm supposed to embrace in order to achieve *Perfect* Me (emphasis on "perfect" is mine). So what about this tension between the command that we be happy and content with who we are and how we look, and the chronic pursuit of perfection (which for me would include some incredible dimples)?

I never got the dimples. I never morphed into a willowy blonde. But I did try to play to what I thought were my strengths.

For years, I thought I had the most *beautiful* feet. They were small and cute and I had the most delightful (albeit stubby) toes. Two toes on each foot were slightly webbed; this was a genetic curiosity I shared with my grandfather and my mother (and my crazy-sweet niece Anne Riley). Despite some inside family jokes about ducks, outstanding swimming ability and my astrological sign (Pisces), I spent more than three decades quietly smitten with my feet. I didn't brag about them (so inappropriate!), but I did take pride in how divine they looked in my Dr. Scholl sandals and teal-blue Candie's. It wasn't until I was dating Brad that I had a cold hard splash of tootsie reality.

We were snuggling on the couch and I asked my sweet future husband to rub my feet. Without hesitation, I presented my feet to him, primed and ready. He quietly got up, went into my bedroom and returned with a pair of socks. "Would you mind putting these on first?" he asked. Undeterred, I sat up and responded, "A foot massage with socks ON? What's the fun in that?" That's when the podiatric intervention happened. Brad sat down and took my hands (not my feet) in his.

"Honey, there is something you need to know. I love you. I love everything about you. But you do not have pretty feet. In fact, despite how much I do love you, I am slightly skeeved out by your feet. Especially your toes. Could you try not to flex them so much?"

I looked at him, speechless. I was not angry, but stunned. Telling me my feet weren't cute wasn't merely an insult, it was an assault on all that I thought right with the world. It was like saying the sky is green and the grass is blue. It didn't compute in my small brain. I knew my Achilles' heel when it came to looks and it was NOT my feet. My teeth are crooked. I have that weird swirly cowlick on my forehead. I have a mole on my chin and am forever battling a unibrow. But skeevy toes and unattractive feet? Never entered my mind. I worked to gently correct such misinformation.

"Oh, sweetie," I countered in a gentle, loving tone. "I'm sorry, but I do have very cute feet. I've had cute feet all of my life. And my twin toes are really quite endearing. Look!" I said this while gazing deeply at my feet, barely noticing Brad turn away slightly when I started flexing my twinned toes.

"Um, no, hon, you really don't." And Brad excused himself to go to the bathroom.

Still not believing it could be true, I started polling family members, childhood and college friends, demanding to know their honest opinion of my feet. The response ensured an emotional roller coaster through the seven stages of grief. Suffice it to say, I now have a very clear appreciation of what qualifies as "attractive feet." And I don't have them.

I'm not bitter, I swear I'm not. Even though I'm talking about it years after the fact, I am at peace with it. In fact, I've come to the conclusion that toes are *not* a fashion accessory. Toes are not meant to be decorated as if they're puppets—with charms, appliqués or rainbows. Toes are not designed to be mascots. A well-manicured foot should say, "My feet are groomed and well maintained. Just like the rest of me." In other words, toes should be a reassuring testament. Less is always, always, *always* more when it comes to feet.

As such, not everyone can wear open-toed shoes. But if you insist on them, then, please, for the sake of Christian Louboutin, buy them in the right size. If one's toes are so long that they hang over the front of the sandal in a griplike fashion—do not buy that sandal. It doesn't fit. Keep on shopping and go up a size—your feet and friends will thank you. The same is true if you have thick ankles and just found a pair of fabulous wedges with an ankle strap on sale—you need to take that very sturdy gait and walk away. Your feet (and ankles) weren't made for that sandal. Ultimately, you need to recognize and play to your strengths, which might reside above your ankle.

All of this is to say that not every appendage and feature is meant to be highlighted, accentuated and glammed, ESPE-CIALLY if you have bunions, or if your toes are nearly as long as your pinky finger. Do people think that a couple of shiny coats of OPI's Mrs. O'Leary's BBQ polish are going to camouflage one toe growing perpendicular to the others?

One of life's great (and hard-learned) lessons is to embrace that which we are, and to accept that which we are not. And I'm not the only middle-aged, slightly disillusioned gal to have figured it out.

My sister-in-law grew up in Saudi Arabia, which seems more startling if you've met her; she has flaming red hair, searing blue eyes, pale ivory skin and a gorgeous smattering of freckles.

Elise is the youngest of four, born to schoolteachers who lived on an American oil base during the heyday of the seventies. She tells stories of leaving the American compound in a burka, as per the legal custom. "I kind of liked it," she once told me, because she was so physically out of place in Arabia that she loved the head-to-toe coverage. It camouflaged the skin that would not tan, the hair that could not be tamed. The athletic frame that did not fit in. In family photos, I can identify her only by her eyes—an astonishing robin's-egg blue. She yearned for the deep, chestnut-brown skin color of the Saudis, coveted their ability to absorb the sun's rays without burning and recognized their deep olive complexions for what they were: a ticket into a world in which she would never belong, despite her best efforts.

Elise daydreamed about a magic potion—part lemon juice, part hair conditioner, part sand—that would erase her freckles forever and allow her to acquire the dark, seamless tan of the Saudis. A tan that would never, ever be part of her DNA. To help along this mythical tan, she oiled her body and lay prone on sizzling sand dunes while the relentless Saudi sun literally blistered her skin. After all, a dark red burn is mighty close to a dark brown tan, she reasoned.

Elise still frets about those blond-red eyelashes and brows, the plight of red hair turning gray and her strong, athletic build. She doesn't see how confident she looks running after her babies on the beach or how much she favors her mother. On occasion she still sees the gawky outsider who burned instead of tanned, who never fit in in a country that had little use for women, much less a freckly, redheaded one. In her forties, like a lot of women, she is still learning to embrace what she's got and let go of what she's not.

And this doesn't just apply to the physical. A queen of to-do lists, high priestess of productivity and manager of many things, including little people, I consider myself a master multitasker. Or I did.

Three summers ago, I was at the beach with my extended family. It was a quaint little family beach that lacked basic amenities like restaurants and a gas station but quietly flouts an expansive beach line and pristine sunsets. The family house sits beachfront, the second-to-last home on a pebbly main street that dead-ends into a beautiful inlet. I grew up going to this beach every summer and loved that, thirty years later, I could lounge on the same beach, feet perched in the same surf, reading some embarrassingly cheesy piece of chick lit. My sister-in-law, still of the alabaster skin, was sporting a two-piece bathing suit that showcased her killer abs. We were keeping track of five kids, all under the age of eleven. When Elise left with her youngest, Charlie, to look for shells, I was left with four, including Anne Riley, my five-year-old cosmic twin of a niece.

Like all moms, I imagine, my mental radar sounded about every fifteen minutes or so and I looked up, scanned the immediate area and took a head count. Initially, Anne Riley wasn't within my scope of sight, but I soon spotted her about a hundred yards away schmoozing with another family under their spacious tent. Like her aunt, Anne Riley is a flaming extrovert and was chatting up some seven-year-old with a cool sand shovel the color of cherries.

"Anne Riley," I said, after I'd captured her and steered her back our way. "You can't wander off without telling me. I didn't know where you were!"

"But, Aunt Char Char, I knew where *you* were." She stared up at me, squinting into the sun. This girl was beyond stinking cute.

We requisitioned a miniature Dora the Explorer beach chair and plopped it next to mine, along with a bag of Goldfish and a juice box. I settled back into my book, eager to learn whether Dare, the hunky private PI, would rescue his love interest from a dishonorable ring of human traffickers. (I know, I'm embarrassed.)

Just as Dare, who has some crazy martial-arts fighting skills, was taking on the drug traffickers in a dark, deserted warehouse, Elise came back with Charlie. "Where's AR?" she asked, after doing her own radar scan. I didn't look up; it wasn't looking good for Dare.

"She's right around here somewhere," I offered, waving my arm in some careless gesture, my eyes never leaving the page. "She snuck away a bit earlier and I got her settled with a snack." I then looked down at the Dora chair and found the crackers and juice box untouched.

Elise continued to scan the beach. "I don't see her. I'm going to walk to the house to see if she went back to use the bathroom."

I dropped my book and started scanning the beach while Elise walked to the oceanfront house. No Anne Riley. Elise returned, calling Anne Riley's name, and then quickly made her way over to the bay side of the beach. No Anne Riley there either.

About then, three giant bubbas came huffing up from the bay. These good ol' boys were shirtless, and unlike Dare, they had a just-rolled-out-of-bed look that indicated not a lotta grooming, not crazy-dirty sex appeal.

To their credit, they did all have their teeth.

"We heard y'all yellin'. Did y'all lose someone?" one asked.

"Yes," blurted Elise. "A five-year-old named Anne Riley. She's about yea high and is wearing a green-and-blue bathing suit."

"We been fishin' on the bay side; she's not over there. But let's help you look."

My mother, in the meantime, had been alerted and was searching the house over again. She was dangling off the porch balcony within desperate earshot. "What can I do?" she called.

One of the bubbas turned to us. "How long's she been gone?"

Elise and I struggled with an answer. We seemed to have lost any sense of time and place. "Maybe twenty minutes," I said. It was a guess.

"Call 911," the bubba yelled toward the porch. I watched my mother's body freeze for a moment, paralyzed by the gravity of the command. She put her head down and turned toward the house to get the phone. Bubba number one took off down a boardwalk at a comfortably urgent jog.

Call 911? We had come to that?

I looked at Elise, and sunglasses couldn't hide the look that passed between us. Elise, the steely, levelheaded investment-banker MBA who married my brother, took a deep breath before she barely whispered, "Okay, Char, what do we do now?"

"You stay right here on the beach. Send the kids to the house with Mom. I'm going to check the other houses—they all look alike. Maybe she wandered into the wrong one and is too scared to move." When Elise left, I marched through the sand to each pastel-colored house, banging on locked doors and boldly walking into empty, unlocked ones. No Anne Riley. I hustled back. My eleven-year-old daughter was nearly mute with fear. Her eyes were as big as the seashells Charlie had collected earlier. Everyone stared at me, numbed by questions that no one had the nerve to ask.

"Look," I told everyone, including Elise. "We are going to find Anne Riley. We are doing everything right. We have people helping us. We called 911. We gave a very detailed description. While I'm worried that she's not with us, I'm not worried that we won't find her."

All of those words were true. Up until that very moment, I believed every single one of them from the very bottom of my heart. But the minute they left my lips, they became lies, lies, lies. And the reality of the situation sank in. I closed my eyes while the nausea and panic washed over me in a tidal wave. I was too panicked to feel guilty. That would come later.

This is what the unimaginable feels like, I thought. It settled on me like a wet, dank towel. Both hot and bone-chilling at the same time.

People wandered up to Elise and me. Murmurings about a lost child—everyone's collective nightmare—had made their way down the beach. "I heard about a missing girl and called 911 from my cell," said one mother. Elise and I looked at each other—I'm not sure we knew cell phones even worked on the beach. Another mother reached out and squeezed Elise's arm in silent sympathy. Minutes passed but it could have been days. One of the bubbas rushed up. I was surprised to see him. I had nearly forgotten about the three heavy, sun-scorched fishermen who were canvassing the beach on our behalf.

"We got word that they found somethin' farther up the beach," one of them said. "Come on."

Found something?

Elise looked around as if searching for invisible arms into which she could fall. Her face stretched in pent-up anguish. "You go," she said. "I need to stay here in case she comes back or if the police come. "

I nod. It had been forty minutes by then, give or take. Bubba number two turned and started to jog, expecting me to follow.

This is where you need to know something.

I don't run. Never have. I am not opposed to running and, in fact, recognize all of the mental and physical benefits of running. My postcollege roommate of five years ran daily. My husband has run in two marathons. His brother, upward of two dozen. I, on the other hand, am a running voyeur. I read books about running, I like to watch people run, and am fascinated by the fact that runners track mileage and change out their shoes every three months or so. Which doesn't mean that I want to do it. Or can.

Having said that, I'm not completely worthless. I am a brisk walker and I can make a mean dent on the elliptical machine at the gym. And when I use my legs (not my back), I can lift heavy things. But I can't run. My lower back hurts. My thighs jiggle and slap at each other like prissy little girls. My stomach rolls around in ways that feel wholly unnatural. Running feels clunky and awkward and my heart feels like it's going to blow out of my chest. Sometimes I'll work a little sprint into my power walk, but I have never, ever by choice run more than a mile in my entire adult life. And now I found myself, at forty-four years old, desperate to run.

I watched Bubba number two clipping down the beach. He had to weigh in at close to 250. He had a fairly sizable beer gut, various and sundry tattoos, reflective NASCAR sunglasses and cutoff shorts. He was shirtless and sweating bullets. He was a hot jogging mess. I took in the scene and fully realized what I had to do.

For the love of Skoal, I thought, if Bubba can run, surely I can, too. And so I started to run. I tried to focus on Bubba's bare feet. I mimicked his gait and kept my head down. I counted my breaths and worked desperately not to vomit. And I considered a quick shout-out to Mercury, the Roman god of speed, to go easy on me as I ran down the beach in search of precious Anne Riley.

People were standing at attention along the way, silently aware of what was unfolding in front of them, with the reverence of a funeral procession. Some looked straight at me. Some turned away. I would have done the same. Who wants to look into the face of someone living out the unthinkable?

I kept running.

It was hot and the heat of the day had cast a hazy glaze over the beach. I tried to stay fixed on Bubba's firm, flat gait, terrified to even glance toward the water. I finally looked up, and I saw the beach patrol ATV driving toward me. It appeared out of focus, like a mirage in the desert. Bubba had stopped. Hands on his knees, he was bent over, catching his breath and talking to the beach patrolman. A patrolwoman, actually. She was petite, with spiky gray hair. Her name was Beth, I would later discover. And while she talked to Bubba, she was gently stroking a tiny little hand that was tucked in hers.

I squinted and looked harder. And tried to run a little faster. The outline of a little person started to form in my line of sight, washed in shades of a blue-and-green one-piece racer-back swimsuit. And before I knew it, I was right there with her.

As suddenly as the nightmare had happened, it was done.

"Hey you, what's going on?" I gently asked, squeezing Anne Riley's other hand. To do anything else at that moment could have resulted in some over-the-top keening that would have caused the poor girl to spend a lifetime in therapy. And likely put me in a straitjacket.

"I needed to rinse off my hands before I had my snack," she replied. She was not crying, but quietly contemplative. She was scared; I could tell by her demeanor. She knew I was, too. Later we discovered that when the beach patrol vehicle approached Anne Riley, the little wayward dynamo had volunteered, "Are you looking for me?"

Elise arrived moments later, the outward epitome of calm. I stepped back as she fell to her knees in front of her daughter and gently wrapped her strong and beautifully freckled arms around her. I turned away. Sweat poured into my eyes and what I thought was a gasp for air turned into a thick sob of release.

Right then, the bubbas surrounded me. All of us were out of breath and speechless, semidelirious with joy and sweet relief. I opened my mouth to thank them, but I was empty. I took off my sunglasses and rubbed my sweaty face with the back of my sandy hand. I just stood there and started crying, wide open like a toddler on the first day of preschool. One of the bubbas gathered me up in his huge arms.

"Come here, sugar," he commanded. "I think this calls for a group hug." And he pulled me in close with the other shirtless, sweaty, tattooed bubbas. I sniffled and cried and pressed my face into a very wet, very hairy and very hot armpit for longer than I care to remember. And it couldn't have mattered less. All four of us huddled together, me and the three nameless bubbas, arms circling each other. I offered up prayers of thanks and I thought about that ridiculously heroic and hunky PI named Dare, the one from my ridiculously inflated summer novel, who managed to save the day, win the girl and save mankind—all before sunset. While Dare was a character in a work of fiction, a figment of someone's imagination, my three bubbas were very real. And just as heroic.

My mother spent the rest of the day in her bedroom with the lights off and a cold compress on her head. Elise sat on the porch, nursing a stiff noontime drink. All of the children, including AR, were safely settled down in front of a movie.

I paced around the kitchen and processed my *Chariots of Fire* moment. Sure, it wasn't pretty—my hair wasn't blowing in the wind and there wasn't some cool symphonic music playing in the background. But I did consider this. I am at peace with my not-very-cute feet, I will never be tall enough to buy pants that don't need alterations, and when I wear bangs I look frighteningly like Joy Behar. I throw a mean dinner party and I can whistle really loudly with my fingers. And I have a manly, generous and gallant trio of unpolished and down-to-earth bubbas who will always remind me that when I really need to run, I can.

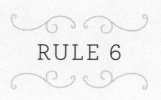

RULE 6

Keep a Stiff
(and Well-Waxed)
Upper Lip

One of my first jobs was at a PR firm in New York, and I was ready to run great lengths to forge a career in the Big Apple. My boss had other ideas. She had jet-black hair cut in delicate, shoulder-length layers, pale porcelain skin that she tempered with bold shades of lipstick and beautiful hands with long, slender fingers. She wore Chanel suits, Ferragamo pumps and strings of pearls. She also smelled lovely—a delicate waft of flowers trailed behind her as she walked the halls. She managed fashion and retail clients, no surprise.

I would have idolized my boss had it not been for the fact that she was the most heinously insensitive and nasty boss on the face of the earth. Often first bosses are. On top of that, she had a squeaky, nasally voice that reverberated down the halls like the screeching sounds of a great horned owl. While I learned a great deal from her—the proper length of one's fingernails, the proper stack of one's heels and the proper way to address Her Majesty the PR Goddess, the most important thing I learned was this: don't ever, ever, ever cry in front of your boss. EVER.

That's what the handicapped stall in the bathroom is for.

I used the handicapped stall on the twenty-fourth floor at 40 West Fifty-seventh Street to scream, to cry and to curse my nitpicky-perfect boss, my unfair client, my abysmal love life and any other woes that needed to be drowned out by industrial flushing sounds. The other benefit to freaking out in the handicapped stall was that the toilet sat quite a bit higher, and for short folks like me, that meant my feet rarely dangled low enough for people to catch a glimpse of who was wailing/flushing in the last stall on the right. (And everyone knows you can ID coworkers by their footwear, am I right?) So, crying in the handicapped stall offered a bit of anonymity and privacy. And time to pull myself together.

Getting and staying pretty at work was a harder task than I had bargained for. After all, when I got out of college, there was a reason that I didn't apply to be a flight attendant, and it didn't have to do with my fear of drowning in miles and miles of endless ocean after floating on a piece of crushed fuselage for seventeen days . . . while wearing polyester. It had to do with small, cramped bathrooms that left little room for sobbing jags, and the fact that I didn't really fit the uniform.

I didn't have to be gorgeous to do my PR job. But I did have to be pulled together on the outside and the inside. And on days with my perfectly coiffed boss breathing down my slightly stained double-breasted linen jacket from an Ann Taylor sale that was in desperate need of a good dry clean, it felt nearly impossible.

That's when I learned that maintaining a stiff upper lip is an essential aspect of decorum. They don't teach that in cotillion class, I can tell you. Rather, it's a lesson that comes through painful self-discovery. I got myself into this job situation, and it was up to me to either survive and thus thrive, or give up and find another job. Neither aspect was appealing, but I had rent to pay. Besides, keeping a stiff upper lip isn't something most of us gals learn postcollege. Usually, it's middle school.

Middle school is undoubtedly where many of us learned how to stay cool under pressure. My friend Michelle remembers the gauntlet of mean girls she had to pass every morning on the way to homeroom. They perched like vultures on the heaters across from their lockers outside their homerooms, ready to pluck away at the already eviscerated innards of their prey with a look, a whispered comment, a raised eyebrow. Michelle learned to keep her head down, her jaw tightly set in a bland smile. Her only goal was to blend in, like a foundation that merges seamlessly with your skin tone.

But often, keeping your head down, your lip stiff and praying to blend in isn't enough. Sometimes, life throws you some serious curveballs that prevent you from keeping a low enough profile. Case in point, my face.

My first two bouts with an MRSA staph infection came at terrible times, but really is there ever a good time to come down with an incredibly antibiotic-resistant staph infection? For those

not in the know, MRSA is a pesky and highly virulent strain of
DEATH that pops up in high school locker rooms and nursing
homes, and if not treated, it can KILL YOU. My initial encounter took root in 2011 the night before a major speaking engagement in another city. I woke up in my hotel room, wandered into
the bathroom, looked in the mirror and screamed. (Actually, it
was more like a low, throaty gasp.) I made my way to the front
desk, got directions to the urgent care and hightailed it over
there, only to find the urgent care wasn't open yet. Fortunately,
the urgent care was connected to the ER, which is always open.
So, with insurance card in hand, I made my first and only
appearance at the ER.

You should know that I have an aversion to the emergency
room. Not because my grandmother always warned me to
NEVER get admitted to the hospital because "they'll kill you
one way or another once you get there." And not because
emergency rooms really are a petri dish of humanity. I have an
aversion to the ER because of my sister-in-law. Apparently, my
fabulously sophisticated, seriously well-educated, impressively
employed sister-in-law LOVES the ER. She has visited at least
a half dozen times since she married into our family. (Only one
trip that I am aware of involved an ambulance.) Nonetheless,
there is great discussion, fanfare and activity around Elise's ER
odysseys and the decisions, ailments and health concerns that
led her to those giant swinging doors to health-care hell. And
while I consider myself to be a connoisseur of drama, I eschewed
any temptation to walk toward those swinging doors, despite
their siren call to me. Trips to the ER seemed so, well, serious.

I left the ER without an official diagnosis, but had two antibiotic prescriptions, a promise of a phone call regarding the
culture, and a pad of gauze taped on my face. My face was
swollen and the infection, which was festering on the lower left
side, near my chin, swelled inward, making my speech thick. I
called my contact at the conference at which I was speaking.

"Hi, Molly, thith is Chawla Mulla," I mumbled. "I've just left
the emergenthee room with an infecthun in my faith. I'm not
thure I can thpeak today."

"Well," she replied crisply. "It's written in your contract that
you cannot cancel without financial penalty, so are you sure this
is what you want to do?"

"I can athure you, Molly, it is NOT what I want do," I said.
"Before we go there, why don't I come to your offith?" And so I
headed to the conference offices, nestled in the back of a giant
convention center. Molly had gathered the troops, including her
two bosses, both female, and both of whom I knew.

I walked in wearing giant dark sunglasses, which I thought
distracted from the gauze bandage the size of Rhode Island
lodged on my chin. What a sad and pathetic notion. I sat down,
shared my story and then pulled off my dressing. I didn't intend
for the gesture to be so dramatic, but it was. All three women
leaned forward and then reared back and took off in the other
direction—they looked like a very pretty version of the Three
Stooges. It was comic.

"Oh, good heavens!" one of the gals in charge exclaimed.
"You can't speak looking like that—it's horrible!"

"Not to mention that no one could understand a word you

said," said the other lieutenant in charge. "For Pete's sake, go home! We'll figure it all out later."

They hurried me out of there, lobbing air kisses from across the room, and running to grab the Lysol and hand sanitizer, I'm sure. I hauled it back to Pretty City, keeping my head down and my giant sunglasses on. Two days later, on a Sunday, I received a phone call confirming my first official MRSA diagnosis. Monday morning I was sitting on the examination table in the office of my young, attentive dermatologist. She changed up my antibiotics and sent me on my way with a firm suggestion that I remember staph infections don't really fall into her wheelhouse, as they're not "skin conditions" per se. She would be happy to address, however, the inevitable scarring.

While I looked worse than I felt at first, it was a good month before I was able to leave my house without a bandage of some sort. This was a real buzzkill, as it was spring, which, as you know, in my Pretty City is always fun.

My first outing after my outbreak was to take my mother to a funky art auction and soiree. I was desperate to get out. I had been holed up in my house for DAYS, and while my infection was still gingerly bandaged, it was under control. I had taken enough oral antibiotics to cripple a moose, so no need to report me to the CDC. To boot, I was freshly showered and swathed in some dressy white jeans, madras wedges and a lovely J. McLaughlin top. I was having a good hair day, too. So I skipped out of the house with my mother and my MRSA, thinking the well-groomed package might help detract from the obvious facial wound and the sizable bandage. Stiff upper lip, indeed!

But it didn't. While the art soiree was packed with pretty people checking out equally pretty art, it wasn't enough to offset the bold questions and covert glances from well-meaning (and not) friends and acquaintances. As we moved from gallery to gallery, nibbling on cheese and fruit and refilling our wineglasses with Chardonnay, my bandage seemed to cast a pall over the pretty evening.

My neighbor told me later, "Everyone kept asking me about your face. But I didn't tell them a thing. I told them if they really wanted to know, to ask you." She said this with a note of pride in her voice. As if I should have congratulated her for not gossiping about an oozing infection "that can kill" (according to medical reports) while I was standing in the same room as she.

That's when I learned that some things go hand in hand with a stiff upper lip and it's a sort of awareness of what's behind one's stiff upper lip. For example, when someone appears in public with a goiter, a cut, a scab or other strange injury, this should be a universal assumption: *it MUST look exponentially better today than it did yesterday. Perhaps I should give this person some props for making the effort.* How do I know this? Because on the day when I finally felt fit enough to debut my MRSA-mottled face to the world, you can bet your favorite pair of skinny jeans that I looked better than I did the day before. But that's not how pretty computes, is it?

The second MRSA infection flamed up the NEXT spring (it's like the Pretty City Fairy simply didn't want me out having fun), again while I was out of town. I was en route to a business meeting at an acclaimed resort in a small village. I checked in to my beautifully appointed room, called my colleagues to confirm my arrival and told them I would be late to meet our client for cocktails, as I just had an *itty-bitty* little medical issue I needed to address. I tried to downplay it at least until I could confirm my condition. But if there was one thing I learned the first time around, it was that these things come on faster than you can burn pine nuts (yes, that fast). Apparently, the MRSA strain of staph is "special" and "doesn't respond" to traditional antibiotics. Sometimes, being special isn't really all that great.

The small village, by the way, is in the middle of NOWHERE and close to NOTHING, including an urgent care. But in keeping with a high-end, luxury resort, they did have an on-site physician . . . who only kept limited office hours, according to the concierge, and was not seeing patients as he was not on property.

I held my breath as the concierge directed me to the (you guessed it) ER. So I made my way to the hospital, took a number and sat in the lobby to ponder how I had lived forty-plus years never darkening the door of an ER and had ended up there twice in as many years. Karmic payback, I imagine, for all of the times I secretly judged those who used the ER to treat non-life-threatening conditions, including my awesome sister-in-law.

Finally, I found myself in a corner of the ER inner sanctum, perched on a gurney, with a shower curtain serving as a door, while a male nurse triaged my condition.

"I thought I could see the on-site doctor at the resort," I inserted as I answered his questions and offered him my five-minute self-diagnosis at no charge. "But he's not on duty today." He noted my surprise.

"That's because he's working the ER shift tonight here at the hospital," said the male nurse. He shot me a grin and added, "In a town this size, you wear a lotta hats."

Indeed. Based on this information, I expected Andy Griffith meets Marcus Welby, M.D. Instead, I got a trim, efficient doc about fifteen years my senior, wearing khakis and a golf shirt.

I told him I thought I had a MRSA staph infection, I presented the protocol from my previous MRSA staph infection, and then stated I would be eternally grateful if he could start me "STAT" on said protocol. The primary reason I was anxious to get up and running on antibiotics that could kill a tribe of African pygmies was that this nasty infection was lodged between my upper lip and nose, kind of like a Madonna beauty mark gone bad. Really, really bad. All the while we discussed why I was visiting the resort, my current vocation as a marketing consultant, his college-aged daughter who attended a prestigious university and aspired to go into marketing, my lovely tenure at UNC and so on. In the end, the doc opted to swab my oozing little beauty mark, test it and get me started on a less aggressive antibiotic until he could confirm it was MRSA. He couldn't be dissuaded and promised to call me on my cell phone when the results came in. I drove back to the resort, changed my bandage, called my colleagues to tell them I'd be there in time for dinner (not cocktails) and hoofed it to the pharmacy in the tiny little village to fill my useless prescription.

Back in my room, I quickly spiffed up and called my colleagues to give them a heads-up. "Hey, I'm on my way," I started out. "You need to know, though, I'm sporting a bit of an issue on my face. It's not all that bad—for now. But I wanted to let you know."

My colleagues graciously urged me along. But the next morning, before our breakfast meeting, I called one and asked her to drop by my room. Between dusk and dawn, "not that bad" had morphed in to "pretty freaky." But I still needed third-party confirmation. Liz knocked, and I quickly ushered her in. Liz is a no-nonsense gal with bright eyes that radiate intelligence and a boho chic style that makes her look younger than she is.

Standing dressed and ready in the sitting area of my charming little suite, I laid it on the line. "I need you to look at me and honestly tell me that this bulging goiter on my face is not only NOT distracting but also NOT utterly repellent, especially in a work environment." She looked at me, eyes wide, and said nothing as she absorbed my words and my face.

"It's not that bad," she finally countered in a flagrant attempt to make me feel better.

"You are telling a bald-faced lie!" I challenged. "Let me put it this way," I continued, attempting some context. "This is not the worst of it. It will get much worse before it gets better."

That was her cue—the polite look frozen on her face melted

away and the real Liz stepped up. "Well, good grief, girl, then you need to get out of here because that is *nasty*—and you're starting to talk funny." Not that again.

I hung in at the meetings another twenty-four hours, though, negotiating through awkward pauses with clients who either pretended they didn't notice, or tried to politely inquire about the glaringly obvious. Finally, I put us all out of our misery and hopped in my car for the five-hour drive back to Pretty City, frustrated, discouraged and annoyed. I was frustrated because they say once you get this infection, you're likely to get it twice, and I hate it to be so predictable. Discouraged because I knew that the worst was still ahead of me. And annoyed because I went all the way to the ER (again) and couldn't get the right meds (again).

On the way home, my cell phone rang.

"Ms. Muller, this is Doctor G. I'm calling to let you know that your test results indicate you do have a MRSA staph infection. I have to admit, I'm surprised."

Really, the doc who works the ER and moonlights at the luxury hotel (or perhaps it's the other way around, as if I care) is surprised?

"Well, guess what, Doc?" I wanted to shout. "I'm not AT ALL surprised that this oozing facial wound is a form of staph that reacts only to a highly specific antibiotic concocted by some witch lady who lives in the hills of Mount Kilimanjaro and adds in a secret pinch or two of eye of newt. Now I have lost TWO days of my life while you practice safe medicine and I tried to entertain clients with this boil on my face. Even better, I'm forty-eight hours late on getting started on the RIGHT horse pills because you didn't trust the patient who offered to get your daughter hooked up with a killer summer internship. In the meantime, I've been taking useless antibiotics that might help clear up acne on a fifteen-year-old but don't come close to clearing up a volcanic infection so pervasive that it leaves SCARS!"

But I didn't say that. I thanked Dr. G for his time and his call and I hung up. And I tried to keep a stiff upper lip, because to do otherwise really made my face hurt. The drive home was interminably long and I went straight to the drugstore (the one with the drive-thru) to fill my new prescription.

The following spring, right on schedule, my THIRD staph infection popped up, on my brow bone. I was living proof that bad things do happen in threes . . . and usually in the spring. I was running a million miles an hour working on a really fun fund-raiser that was finally coming to fruition. I would NOT be waylaid by another infection, I told myself as I looked in my triple-magnifying mirror for the telltale signs that were there in the form of a red, inflamed, throbbing cyst.

The only good thing that happened after my first two staph infections (besides the fact that they finally went away) was a referral from my sweet, creamy-complexioned dermatologist to a doctor who "specializes in these things." For the record, do you know what kind of doctor specializes in staph infections? An ID doctor. ID as in Infectious Diseases. Do you know who goes to an ID doctor—besides people like me with nasty-gross staph infections on their faces? People with INFECTIOUS DISEASES! I'm not sure why this didn't occur to me until I was sitting in the waiting room surrounded by literature with titles like "Living with HIV" and "Loving a family member with AIDS." In the reception area of the ID practice, the nurses sat behind glass windows and asked you to slip your insurance card and payment through a little hole. It was like a will-call window for infected people.

But at least I was in a marginally better place when MRSA number three hit. I was home, for one—no need for an ER run in a strange city. And two, I had Dr. M, the ID doctor for the famously infected, on speed dial. I called on a Sunday and was there when the doors opened on Monday morning. As I slipped my paperwork to the receptionist through the little portal, I was feeling cautiously optimistic that this would be an easier road than before.

"Oh, good Lord! That looks HORRIBLE!"

That's exactly what Dr. M announced as he BACKED AWAY from me as I primly perched on the examination table in the ID examination room. He looked repulsed and, if I wasn't mistaken, a little green. Aside from my little "facial situation," I was show-ered, well groomed and sporting makeup and jewelry. In other words, I was trying.

"Um, Dr. M, you're an ID doctor," I said slowly. "Aren't you used to this kind of thing?"

"Well, sure," he responded in his slightly nasal Midwestern accent, never taking his eyes off mine. He held his hand up as if he wanted to touch my face, but couldn't bring himself to actu-ally do it. "But this looks really bad. I mean, have you seen it?"

Really? Had I SEEN this alien infection that had taken root

on my brow bone? What is this, some kind of quack comedy routine? "Yes, I've seen it. That's why I'm here, Doctor M. I need to be on the way to recovery in forty-eight hours—I have a HUGE fund-raising event on Wednesday with five hundred of my closest friends, and not only can I not miss it, I need to look presentable. So let's roll."

"Well," he said while he continued to squint at my "situation," "I'm thinking we should do some IV antibiotics for the next few days and then we'll see what happens."

I rubbed my hands together. Quick diagnosis, quick action— IV antibiotics have to be better than oral meds, right? I liked his style. "All right, then. When do I start?"

"How about right now?" he said. "I'll walk you back to the IV room and introduce you to Tammy. She'll get you hooked up." And he meant that literally. Tammy got me hooked up and Dr. M came back swathed in rubber gloves and covered my eye in a giant gauze bandage.

While all of this was a bit unexpected, I liked the sense of urgency and the level of care. I called work to tell them I would be late, texted Brad that things were moving along quite smoothly with my treatment and reminded myself to bring my Kindle when I came back tomorrow. The next morning, I came and went through the same routine. I checked in with the reception gals hermetically sealed behind the glass wall, walked back to the IV room and checked in with Tammy. She seated me in one of the dozen IV chairs, wheeled an IV stand over, grabbed a pillow on which to prop my arm and sat down on a rolling stool with her stash of "magic" potions and her usual bag of tricks. The day before, the IV room had been all but empty. But that day, there was a little more action. An older, attractive black woman sat reading her *Guideposts*. A gray-headed grandmother with a crocheted blanket over her lap sat dozing. A few others were sprinkled in the mismatched treatment chairs. The IV room sat at the back of the building and was directly accessible from an outside entrance—I learned later that the outside entrance was more wheelchair accessible. After day two of my IV, I popped into Dr. M's office, per his request.

"SOOOO, whaddya think, Dr. M?" I asked. "Are things looking up? Think I can swing my big event tomorrow?" He peeled off the bandage he'd applied the day before and his brows knitted. "Ewwww," he said, peering closely with that strange expression again on his face. "This is not looking good." And he turned to carefully throw the bandage in a trash can plastered with giant red warning labels about contamination, disease and pending doom.

I have to say that Dr. M's "bedside" vibe of squeamish third grader was bumming me out. But I was even more bummed when he announced that I needed more than two days of IV antibiotics. I tried to rally. "That's okay," I responded. "Can I swing by after my event tomorrow, around one or so?"

"I'd really rather you come first thing in the morning so I can check you out and change your bandage." The man was totally stepping on my fancy-luncheon-with-five-hundred-of-my-cute-friends buzz, but I agreed.

The next morning my fancy-luncheon-with-five-hundred-of-my-cute-friends buzz had morphed into *for the love of chicken salad gently placed on Bibb lettuce, what happened to my eye?!*

I did not stare into my triple-magnifying mirror, as it was hard to look into my triple-magnifying mirror with only ONE EYE! The other was swollen shut, and the infection in my brow was protruding over my eye like a strange stalactite. My giant sunglasses wouldn't even sit on my face, much less cover the stalactite. I turned to Brad, the king of understatement, who stood at the bureau and tied his tie. He cast me a worried look. "Yeah, hon, I don't think you're going to your luncheon today."

My false optimism and bravado fell away as I realized that my IV treatments were not some magical elixir that would allow me to outrun what I knew to be a long and arduous and very icky recovery, requiring people to lance, drain, squeeze and "excavate" (I swear to you, that's the word they used) things on my face. That despite my having avoided the ER and ducking a false start on the wrong meds, this was going to run a similar course. A course that did not include my attendance at a series of fundraising events at which I had key responsibilities. A course that would impact my work schedule and my ability to just "stay on top of my business," as we like to say in my family.

Before I headed out to see Dr. M and Tammy, I called two girls whom I was hosting at the luncheon. I left a message of profuse apology for one, gave her details on her table placement and encouraged her to go and have fun. I called my other friend Cyndee, and she answered. After my abbreviated version of "Scar Wars," Cyndee announced, "Why don't I just go with you to the doctor?" I protested. My first two days solo at the IV clinic had gone just fine. Brad hadn't gone with me. I'm not sick. Besides, Cyndee didn't know what she was getting into.

"The only reason I was going to the luncheon was to be with you," she reasoned. "Besides, it's raining, I don't have anything to wear and I feel fat today." Well, she had me there. "I don't have anything to wear and I feel fat" are the universal distress signals for women everywhere. Morse code we all understand and, by duty, cannot refuse to accommodate.

"All right," I said. "It will be nice to have company. I'll pick you up—you're on my way."

"Where is your doctor?" she asked.

"Oh, you'll see," I responded ominously, and hung up.

I called three girls in charge of the fund-raiser to tell them I had a medical emergency and could not attend to my assigned duties at the luncheon. One of the girls picked up.

"Hi, Barb, it's Charla."

I started out: "I'm really sorry to do this, but I can't come today. I've had a little medical issue come up."

"Beg your pardon? Did you say you aren't coming today? At all?" Insert very long and awkward pause.

Well, this was going to go well. I outlined all the things I had done and all the things I needed to do and tried to assure her that all my duties would be handled. At least I tried to assure her, but I'm pretty sure she hung up in the middle of my update.

I picked up Cyndee. She got in the car, turned to me and arched an eyebrow. "Wow, you look like a mummy. Is all that gauze really necessary?"

That's the great thing about Cyndee—the girl is bluntly honest and has little patience for the puny or sickly, as she is rarely either. She ranks high on the efficiency scale and low on the drama scale. She wears her blond hair short short and fluffy and simply finger-dries it after every shower. She is so low maintenance and on top of her stuff that she requests that people DON'T bring her casseroles and such after major life events. In fact, she popped out three nearly ten-pound babies without missing a beat. If Cyndee could have delivered those babies at home while vacuuming and playing Words with Friends, she would have been a happy camper.

At a stoplight, I slid my bandage down to give her a peek. "Hmm," she said. "It doesn't look all that bad." I tried to give her the stink eye, but my oozy eye was swollen shut.

Cyndee had to wait in the reception area at Dr. M's office, which was just fine by her as she was as fascinated as I by this whole medical underworld of infectious diseases. She sat there, people-watched and played Words with Friends. Before I could offer up "staphylococcus" as a real showstopper, I was ushered back to see Tammy and then on to Dr. M.

"Well, Doctor," I said as I shimmied onto the examination table with a cotton ball tucked in the crook of my arm, "Tammy and I have become fast friends, but my eye is worse than it was yesterday. And what in the world does one wear with white gauze and medical tape this time of year?" I plied him with good humor and pluck in an effort to counterbalance my growing concern.

This time when Dr. M peeled back my bandage he was

unusually quiet. His jolly demeanor and throaty giggle (he giggles, I can't explain it, but he does) were replaced by serious concentration. That big smart head of his, stuffed full of education from Vanderbilt and Emory, was in overdrive. After peering into my face, he stood up and leaned against the wall with his hands behind his back and looked at me.

"This doesn't look good," he started. I was smart enough not to offer some quippy response about looking good *in any way, shape or form* in this condition. "The IV antibiotics don't seem to be working yet, and the infection is getting more intense. I'm concerned that the infection is going to spread into your eyelid, which has tissuelike skin, or behind your eye. We need to lance and excavate the infection area." See? That word "excavate" again. As if my face was some prehistoric archaeological site.

"Okay," I responded, not sure of any other appropriate answer. It wasn't like I was going to shop around for a second opinion or decide that I was just not in the mood for an archaeological dig in my face that day. "What do you have to do?"

"Well, that's the thing," he said. "The infection is in a very vulnerable place, right above your eye, on your brow bone. I'm not the best person to do the procedure. I'm going to call over to a plastic surgeon at the eye practice and see if he can do it."

"Okay," I responded again. "When?"

"Right now. Do you have someone to drive you there and then take you home?" he asked. There was no mistake in reading between those lines. Then he hustled out of the exam room to make some calls. I texted Cyndee, who was two rooms over, and asked her how much time she had this morning.

All the time you need, friend, she texted back. I threw on my sunglasses, which sat sidesaddle on my face, stiffened my upper lip and headed into what was next.

As I was called back to the exam room at the ophthalmology practice, Cyndee asked if I needed her to come along. "Do you want to come along?" I asked.

"Not really, but I felt the need to offer."

That's my girl—all business with a dash of thoughtfulness. "I'm good. Just enjoy your Words with Friends and I'll try to be quick." After all, I told myself, I'm not that sick.

Dr. P was bald as a Ping-Pong ball. As I sat in the examination chair, I marveled at how shiny his head was and wondered if he polished it every day. Dr. P was not a plastic surgeon but an ophthalmologist—but both kinds of doctor cut things, I reasoned. Not exactly what Dr. M had ordered, but infected beggars can't be choosers, I thought, and made myself comfortable.

"Do you do these procedures often?" I asked as he busied himself with all of his equipment, laying it all out in an orderly fashion.

"Well, when I was in residence in Texas, I saw MRSA infections all the time. All the Mexicans had them." Wow, how to respond?

He proceeded to put one of those dental bibs around my neck and then put one over my face. The one on my face had a little porthole cut out so he could get to my eye. "But do you do these procedures often?" I pressed.

"Not many," he admitted as he held a giant syringe of numbing solution above me. My little face bib was rising and falling as I puffed and tried to breathe.

He moved toward me, his arm still raised high over my head. The needle twinkled under the direct light from the examination lamp. It was like a scene from a bad horror flick. "Now, this is going to hurt," he said. "Are you ready?" He seemed uncertain and hesitant. Which made me uncertain and hesitant. He brought the needle closer, then stopped.

"Are you ready?" he asked again, his hand poised in midair. Still very uncertain and still very hesitant. I'm staring at the needle, strangely aware that this really did feel like a scene from a bad horror flick. He started again.

"I'm going to do it now, okay? So tell me when you're ready because this is really going to be uncomfortable. Seriously. Are you ready?" Okay, maybe a Monty Python riff on a bad horror flick.

My little face bib started flapping in the wind as my breathing quickened. "Yes, do it already," I croaked, and white-knuckled the chair. My hypothesis that ophthalmologists didn't do this sort of thing very often proved true when he dug that needle around in my brow bone until numbing solution streamed down my face like tears.

"There," he said as he disposed of the needle. "That needs to numb up. I'll be back in a few minutes."

"Take your time," I gasped as I tried to catch my breath. Fifteen minutes later, he came back, ready to dig into my numbed eyelid. It was excruciating, and was made even more excruciating by his heavy hand and utter uncertainty. For every minute that went by, I wondered if this torture could possibly last another.

Finally, I yelled uncle.

"I'm sorry, I know you're not done, but I need a minute," I whispered from underneath my facial bib. I had maintained an incredibly stiff upper lip and I needed a private moment. The man didn't walk, but rather sprinted from the room.

And I burst into tears.

I know, I'm a weenie. So sue me. But after two C-sections and some heavy-duty dental work in my thirties (including a root canal while thirty-eight weeks pregnant), I had struck the mother lode—an eye doc trying to excavate a facial staph infection in an exam room intended for eye dilation. And where the heck was a nurse? I wanted to know. Wasn't there supposed to be someone here to witness this gruesome scene or scream for help if something went horribly wrong? It wasn't like I could reach the giant red emergency button from my chair.

So I sat in the chair and just boohoo'd. I lifted the facial bib so I wouldn't get snot on it. I thought it was the least I could do. About ten minutes later, I had pulled it together. Dr. P knocked on the door, entered and finished the very messy job he had started, which included creating three "exit" sources for the infection. Apparently, this is common procedure that allows the infection to come out of predetermined "lances" in the skin rather than "bursting" through it (which would be bad). He packed the excavation area with medicated gauze, covered it with an eye patch, wrote me a prescription for a painkiller and somberly insisted I get it filled ASAP.

That was rich. The man had just dug a hole into my brow bone, stuffed it with chemical-laced cotton, graciously left me with three exit wounds—all with the finesse of a lumberjack—and he thought I was NOT going to take the freakin' painkillers? He left the room and I cast about trying to gather up my belongings and my wits.

Dazed, I silently walked out of the room and found myself in a retail area that sold eyeware—pretty frames by Kate Spade and Calvin Klein dotted delicate glass shelves. I was confused until it dawned on me where I was. Turning around to get my bearings, I saw my image in a mirror. My face and neck were splotchy and red from crying. My hair was smushed flat from quietly writhing in the examination chair. A quarter of my face was bandaged and another quarter was swollen from the infection. I was a complete wreck. I took a deep breath and went to find Cyndee.

"Hey," she said as I approached, slipping her phone in her handbag, collecting her things and giving me a gentle once-over. "That took a while, didn't it?" I nodded catatonically. She accurately assessed that I was on the brink and so ushered me to the checkout area, where a girl asked if I minded if she put on rubber gloves before she handled my paperwork. Whatever.

It was then that Cyndee kicked into highly productive, take-no-prisoners and take-charge mode. She gave the girl in the checkout area the evil eye (since I couldn't), steered me straight out the door, gingerly plucked my keys from my purse and got me settled into the passenger seat of my own car, all the while distracting me with inane, good-natured chatter. She drove me to the drugstore to get my Oxycontin. She called Brad to update him. She drove me home, got me inside and made sure I was comfortably dosed and on the coach. She stayed until Brad got there. She then carried on with Brad what I thought at the time was mindless conversation but realized later was actually laced with subtle but important details he likely needed to know.

I had no idea that I had arrived home about the time the luncheon with five hundred of my girlfriends wrapped up. But I did glance up at the one girlfriend who stood in front of me, let go of that stiff upper lip and mumbled teary and weary words of incredible gratitude.

I would come to be a part of the little IV clinic community after that. For twelve days, I fell into a rhythm. It was a forced pace that I couldn't accelerate and simply had to embrace. I drove myself to the clinic, Kindle in hand, checked in with Tammy, smiled and nodded at a few familiar faces and looked for my favorite seat. Like church, it was a quiet, almost reverent place. Patients at an ID IV clinic weren't having all that much fun and many were praying for the best, I would come to find out. Also like church, everyone had a favorite seat, the one with the preferred view, close enough to the action or far away enough for comfort. The space where a wheelchair would best fit, or the chair that one could access with crutches. I learned quickly which seats were NOT open for grabs—namely the La-Z-Boy recliner. That was a coveted seat and one I was happy to avoid. Only really sick people sat in the La-Z-Boy for their IV transfusions. And that wasn't me, of course.

One morning, Tammy rolled over on her little stool with wheelies, ready to start.

"Girl, you are black-and-blue all over!" she exclaimed under her breath as she firmly patted the inside of my arm looking for a good vein. "All of these veins are shot. I sure hope I can find a good one today."

I stilled. "What do you mean, you HOPE you can find a good one today?"

"All these are shut down, doll, they won't hold the IV needle," Tammy said. "You really should have a port."

Port? What's she talking about a port? I thought to myself. I'm not THAT sick.

But Tammy kept up her lamenting and her baby slaps up and down my arms until I very nearly grabbed her with both hands by her nurse smock, the one decorated with fish (as her son was an aspiring professional bass fisherman), wheeled her close enough that I was totally up in her junk and yelled, "So help me, Tammy, I don't care if you have to shoot me up between my toes, but you will find a vein in this body and you will insert that needle and you will start that IV bag. Now." But I didn't. Because I wasn't all that sick. And the IV clinic was not a place to make a scene. It was a bit like church, after all.

Instead I sweetly suggested she try the back of my hands.

"Oh, hon, those little veins are so tiny," Tammy said as she softly rubbed one of my hands between hers. "I'll have to use a butterfly needle. You'll be here twice as long 'cuz that fluid can only drip-drop into those little veins. And law, it's just going to beat up your hands, they'll be covered in bruises that you can't cover like you can the ones on your arm."

Jeez, I felt like a junkie at a drug spa. Such gentle care and attention.

"And you can't move neither, darlin', these needles are so tender, any little move can pull them out."

"Tammy," I pleaded. "Right now I've got nothing but time. And I swear on my grandfather's favorite fishing lure, I will not move. Please."

From that day on, Tammy butterflied one hand or the other while I sat as still as a statue and the antibiotic dripped and dropped. And law, it did take forever. But I caught up on my reading—distracting, mindless and cheesy romance novels where the hero and heroine end up happy, healthy and ALIVE. I quietly kibitzed with the other IVers. I learned more about Tammy's family. I listened to music on my iPhone. I texted Brad that I was doing great, no worries. I discovered that Dr. M recently had won a car in a school raffle. And I called my mom. A lot. My mother LOVES medical "situations," so my whole MRSA drama was right up her alley.

One day, I sat next to an older gentleman whom I had seen there before. Like me, he sported an eye bandage. "Looks like you and I have something in common," I said in an effort to drum up some conversation while I remained statue still.

"Yes," he responded with a sly smile and in a thick European accent. "But I suspect you have an eye under yours," he said.

I smiled sheepishly. "Yes, sir, I do have an eye under mine."

"I've been wearing mine since I lost my eye thirty years ago," he offered. His other eye crinkled with a wistful look. "But every day we wake up on the right side of the dirt is a great day, don't you agree?"

I did indeed agree. Despite my eye patch, despite passing my co-pay through a hole in a glass window, despite my bruised hands and arms, despite the fact that the only human touch I had received for the last dozen days was from a medical provider wearing rubber gloves, I totally and unequivocally agreed.

Not only was I waking up on the right side of the dirt, I had an eye under all that padding. In fact, I had a veritable junkyard—medicated packing materials, a Band-Aid or two, gauze, medical tape—all topped off by a gauze bandage the size of a preemie diaper and an eye patch. At first, Dr. M was the only one who changed the dressing, but then I got in the game because I really needed to shower. So I learned to change and to drain daily, sometimes more. My bathroom would be festooned with all sorts of used and discarded medical materials. After each changing-of-the-bandages session, I would sweep all the contaminated medical debris into a plastic grocery bag, cinch it shut and take it directly to the garbage can outside. Do not pass go. Do not collect $200. I would then circle back to douse my countertop, cabinets, floor (and the rest of my body) in rubbing alcohol.

One afternoon after work, I mindlessly started deconstructing my layers of dressing. The process had become rote, much like flipping through the mail on the counter. As I peeled off the layers that included that day a waterproof Band-Aid and thumbed through a pile of catalogs, I heard a strange ripping sound. Puzzled, I looked down at the Band-Aid in my hand and saw what looked like a little caterpillar. I was alarmed and my fingers flew to my forehead, searching for my eyebrow like a blind person trying to read Braille. I couldn't find it, feel it, read it. It wasn't there. I had ripped off two-thirds of my eyebrow with a waterproof Band-Aid.

I tried to keep a stiff upper lip on that one, girls, I really did. But it was just too much and I was too tired. My ongoing struggle with facial hair starting at the age of twelve—all the waxing, the plucking, the shaving (yep, you read that right) and the threading—was the perfect emotional backdrop for the moment I accidentally ripped out hair that I actually liked, needed and intended to keep.

I didn't burst into tears like I had in Dr. P's office. I just shut my eyes as I quietly mourned my lost eyebrow. My daughter, who had wandered into the kitchen and watched this silent drama unfold, kept assuring me it would grow back and that she would gladly give me one of hers. Instead, I drew one on every morning and then covered it with a patch. It didn't matter that no one could see the eyebrow I drew, I still did it. Kind of like wearing nice underwear under your interview suit. No one knows but you. It was a matter of principle.

One day, my friend Julianne called me as I was leaving the IV clinic.

"Darling," she cooed. "I'm calling to confirm you're sitting at our table on Saturday night for the party." Though it was not my "Oscar year," this was yet another part of the fund-raising event I had worked on for the better part of a year. Alarms went off in my head. The gala had unceremoniously fallen off my radar, bumped by daily doc appointments and an unexplained world shortage of medical gauze.

While I had a superfab vintage dress ready to wear (finally I was getting into the groove of what looked good), I was still sporting some significant drainage and swelling. And don't forget my needle tracks and missing eyebrow. In other words, there was still a lot of ugly going on.

"And before you say no," she countered, as if reading my mind, "I want you to come by my house. I'm whipping you up a little couture eye patch to go with your dress."

Having Julianne offer to whip up a custom eye patch to match my dress was like having Ina Garten offer to come by your house to whip up a little dinner. Julianne is a hip, talented gal with a keen and unfailing eye for all things chic. She is also busy, focused and, like many of us, always on the go.

I was honored and very touched. And I'll admit, I got a bit verklempt. I had been shuttling between home, work and the IV clinic, sporting a SINGLE eyebrow. I needed a lift, and it had come in the form of an incredibly thoughtful gesture from a dear person.

The day of the gala, I dropped by Julianne's house with my dress. A room off her kitchen serves as a studio, dressing room and all-purpose holding room for her notions. Drawers full of ribbons, buttons, fabrics and all sorts of pretty things. I brought along an eye patch from the drugstore to use as a pattern. It was bulky and ill-formed.

"Surely we can do better than this," she determined, and tossed the patch aside to start on her own version. Julianne started to clip, sew and create—entering into a creative zone that was fascinating to witness. A few hours and a few samples later, I had in my hand a chic, midnight-blue suede eye patch with leather strips. It was awesome.

Later that evening, I took a long, hot shower, blew out my hair and slipped on my vintage pool dress with rich florals. I carefully penciled in my eyebrow, gingerly covered it with a NON-waterproof bandage, donned my eye patch and dabbed concealer on my IV marks. I glammed up my good eye with a dramatic fake eyelash and some heavy shadow (a little intentional irony for anyone who cared to notice). I took a deep breath and walked into the den to present to Brad.

He looked up from reading his iPad. I smiled nervously. His face burst into a huge grin. "Honey, you look remarkable! I mean it—you are rocking that eye patch." I exhaled a huge sigh of relief. Brad had been quietly attentive throughout this ordeal, but from a distance. It was partly by design—I insisted he sleep in our guest bedroom and shower in the guest bath for fear I might contaminate him. But it was also because he understood that the more he fretted and fussed, the more serious this would all seem—to both of us. There was an unspoken need for us to simply muscle through it all, chins up. The dress, the eye patch and an evening out with friends marked the end of the worst. I grabbed my party clutch as he guided me out of the door.

We arrived at the event. Cute young waiters in Lilly Pulitzer ties met us in front of the club, bearing trays of colorful drinks. Couples strolled across the lawn—pretty women with beautifully arranged hair and fabulous florals that reeked of Palm Beach chic. Photographers circled the group like seagulls, waiting to snatch up a picture like an abandoned bread crumb. My clever eye patch, with its hint of glamour, seemed to put most people at ease. I didn't look sick or injured. And while I skillfully skirted the photographers, I apparently looked healthy enough not to raise the proverbial, if you will, "eyebrow." We ate dinner with Julianne, her husband and two other couples. We danced to live music and we cheered and clapped when Julianne won the raffle for a colorful Lilly Pulitzer beach cruiser—a testament to the power of good karma.

All wasn't perfect. There was the über-glam gal who semi-collided with me on the way to the bathroom. As she brushed past me she exhaled a pointedly rude comment under her breath. She thought I didn't hear, but I did. After all, when one sense is compromised, the others are heightened. So I gave her the evil eye with my one good, highly styled, lushly lashed eye.

I didn't mention the incident to anyone, especially Brad, because it was an incredibly fun evening and it would just have upset him. In a way, he was keeping a stiff upper lip of his own as he gently cajoled and encouraged me during those long weeks of IV needles and his long exile to the guest bedroom. Later that evening, Brad told me, "Honey, you were amazing. There is not anyone I know who would have been able to pull that off like you did." I'm not sure that this is true. I think I have a few girl-friends—Cyndee, Julianne, Elise, Suzanne—who could have stepped up and stepped out just like I did.

Months later, I ran into one of my dinner companions from that evening. A mutual friend started to introduce us.

I interrupted her. "We've met before. We had dinner together at the gala."

He cocked his head, tried to place me but couldn't. I decided to help him out and covered my right eye with my hand. "Remember now?" I said with a grin.

"I totally remember!" he chimed in with a big smile. "I didn't recognize you without your eye patch!"

What's funny is that I wasn't memorable because of my wit, my funky vintage dress, my stylishly coiffed hair, my legendary dinner-party chatter or even my volunteer résumé. I was memorable because I tried to gild a really ugly situation with a killer suede eye patch designed by a fabulously dear and stylish friend. And it worked. In retrospect, I realized that we often keep a stiff upper lip because of what we don't want others to see—hurt, humiliation and embarrassment. But just as important are those times when we keep a stiff upper lip in order to determine, deep inside ourselves, what we're made of. The eye patch was my own personal testament that pretty doesn't just take practice; on occasion it requires some guts.

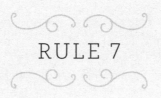

RULE 7

Social Graces Are
the Secret Weapon of
the Pretty and the Plain

Years before my staph-infection odyssey, I was having a glass of wine with my friend and then-neighbor Eve. We were sitting on stools in her kitchen, noshing on cheese and nuts while the kids ran around upstairs and the husbands caught up on whatever things husbands find interesting. Eve's fraternal-twin daughters were about nine or ten at the time, a year younger than my daughter. We were swapping tales of bad teachers, painful home-work projects and elementary school social angst. Which for one of Eve's daughters included a "first crush" on a classmate. When her daughter popped into the kitchen that day, Eve asked her about her crush.

"Mommy," she said, "when I look at Trey, it burns my eyes."

Don't you just love it? It didn't matter if he opened the door to the lunchroom for her, slipped her an oatmeal raisin cookie from his football-shaped lunch box or saved her a seat on the afternoon bus (none of which he did)—she was blinded by his blond hair and green eyes and lopsidedly perfect grin. Trey could be a total third-grade stooge and it wouldn't matter. Like many distractingly good-looking people, basic manners and appropriate behavior simply aren't taken into account.

But what about the pretty plain? Those of us who don't waltz through life with a hall pass of beauty that blinds others to our faults? We require a bit of social finesse to make things easier—for us, and everybody else. Evelyn Waugh summed it up: "Manners are especially the need of the plain—the pretty can get away with anything." Never have truer words been spoken. Fabulously beautiful people behaving badly are everywhere, and we can't seem to turn away.

The veneer of good looks, good grooming and good genes can forgive myriad sins—including boorish behavior and an appalling lack of manners. But for a southerner, pretty or plain, good graces rank up there with a breakfast casserole, well-polished silver and the sacred Easter dress. At the core is the blindingly simple concept of "others first." Standing in the back of the buffet line at the family reunion. Serving yourself a chicken leg (white meat is for the adults) and quietly dining at the kids' table in the sunroom. Sitting in the backseat of the car—not because the front seat airbag would crush anyone under five feet, but because elders always ride shotgun. This is just how it is.

And while putting others first was rooted in our favorite church hymns, it was really about putting adults ahead of children in all things that didn't cause bodily damage or emotional harm. And each generation learned and endured because they knew the day would come when they went through the buffet line first, sat at the head of the table, helped themselves to all the white meat they could manage and rolled home fat and happy in the front seat of their 1982 Ford station wagon. And if that day didn't come? Well, in the South there is more than enough squash casserole for us all.

Now I'm training my own two children, not only in the art of "others first" but also the dying art of "ma'am" and "sir." I've had many "character development conversations" with my son and they usually go one way.

"Son?"

"Huh?"

"Son?"

"Yeah?"

"Son?" I persist, waiting for the right answer.

"Yes?" So close.

Nearly there, I feel it.

"Yes, ma'am?"

At last, the two words that are the keys to the kingdom of manners in my book.

"Could you please come downstairs for dinner?"

"Yes, ma'am."

How sweet it is.

While manners and social graces are part of the cultural foundation in my neck of the woods, I am of the firm opinion these critical requisites make the entire world go round, not just my hemisphere. Because at the heart of good manners and social graces lies the core truth of putting others first and making do with what is served, given and offered. And I'm of the opinion that it's my job as a parent to teach my children that the world is not one big all-you-can-eat buffet.

One of my best pals, Suzanne—she of cute summer sandals and sport cover-ups—used to live in Pretty City before she married the man of her dreams, followed him to Harvard Business School and then settled in a New Jersey hamlet to raise three very bright kids. We take turns visiting each other, intent that our kids will grow up knowing one another despite the weird accents (on both sides) and unhandy geography. So a few summers ago, it was Suzanne's turn to visit me. We were buzzing around town, spending equal time enjoying the heat and avoiding it. That day, we had been out shopping and the kids were home hanging out. We agreed to stop on the way home and grab some Chick-fil-A.

Now, this may come as a surprise, but 80 percent of the menu at Chick-fil-A is chicken. Not burgers, not hot dogs, not roast beef. Chicken. Now, they have lots of ways to order the chicken—filet sandwich, nuggets and strips. Again, this may come as a surprise, but the chicken filet and the chicken nuggets and the chicken strips all taste pretty much the same. 'Cuz they're all chicken. No need to check in with my kids—it's a sure thing that I'll come home with some variation of (you guessed it) chicken.

In the meantime, Suzanne called her kids to take their orders. In fact, she drew a rubric on the back of her checkbook so that she could track their preferences. When she couldn't answer a menu question or confirm a preference, she volunteered to call back once we hit the menu screen. I found this fascinating. The whole reason drive-thru restaurants EXIST is that they're easy and simple. Drive up. Order chicken. Throw in fries. Try a milk shake. Drive home. Don't forget ketchup. Oh, you prefer Polynesian sauce mixed with equal parts ranch dressing? Well, by all means, let me turn back posthaste to get those little packets of tasty goodness.

When your kids have to "make do" with a chicken sandwich instead of chicken nuggets, and a Sprite instead of lemonade, and a vanilla milk shake instead of an Oreo one, you are honing a tiny smidgen of their life skills. When kids can "make do" without giving you the stink eye, running to their room to pout or launching into a twenty-minute dissertation on why you suck as a parent, then you've given them a real gift. Now, Suzanne's kids did none of this, as all three are really good kids and she is a great parent, but she sure spent a lot of time managing their "special orders" that all ended up tasting like . . . chicken.

Which made her consider that there will come a time when our kids won't get exactly what they ordered in that big drive-thru window called life and they might just have not only to make do but to do it in front of a boss, a spouse, a teacher or other people who won't pat them on the back and tell them it's okay, they can circle back later and get their Polynesian sauce mixed with ranch dressing. Lots of life is not only making do but being a good sport about it. I've come to view a visit to Chick-fil-A as an education in character building and graciousness.

As adults, we're not exempt from character building and graciousness. In fact, sometimes it's harder to recognize and embrace the moments when God, the universe or our spouse, best friend or boss is trying to teach us and hone us. Again, gracious behavior requires some social finesse and certainly some manners.

Much like my weekend at the beach with my friend Cyndee, nearly a decade ago. What started out as a casual weekend at my parents' beach house playing cards and drinking wine morphed into a battle of skills and heavy debate on what constitutes a real competitor.

We sat on the back porch dealing out hand after hand of gin rummy and, when the husbands were around, spades. Cyndee smoked a cigarette or two, I noshed on snacks and sipped on wine. Bruce Springsteen and U2 played in the background. And over the course of the afternoon, we both were pushed to the brink. If I misplayed as her partner and we lost, she was sure to let me know, and I was affronted. If I misplayed as her opponent and she won, she let me know, and I was affronted. She was insufferable and I was annoyed. We spent another breezy afternoon doing the same thing. This time, Cyndee soundly beat me, hand after hand, in gin rummy. She was loudly crowing and I was silently seething.

But I hung in there and slowly the tide started to turn.

"Wow, you've been getting some really good cards," she commented as I reshuffled and prepared to deal another hand. I caught the barely perceptible snark in the comment and volleyed back.

"So, what you're saying is that when you win, it's skill of play, and when I win, it's lucky cards?" I challenged. I had spoken a truth that she didn't want to admit—she thought she was a better player and we both knew she thought it.

As explanation for her abrasive competitive banter and play, she threw out, "Well, you know, I'm just one of those people who just really likes to win."

As if people who are gracious losers and generous winners don't like to win all that much, while people who "really like to win" are exempt from the normal standards of sportsmanship and conduct. In other words, Cyndee is a cutthroat competitor, as evidenced by her behavior as a winner and a loser. And I am clearly a milquetoast of a competitor and must not care all that much whether I win or lose since I work to do both with a modicum of low-grade hostility masked by decorum.

Which means that people who really like to drink can be boors at parties, overstay their welcome and insult the hostess on their way out the door. "Well, you know, you really should invite me back anyway. I'm just one of those people who just really likes to drink."

I later decided that Cyndee needed to choose. She couldn't be a smug winner AND a sore loser. Ideally, she would be neither, but at the very least, she could only be one. And she could work on the other. Because part of the art of social graces is that they often require discipline and practice. If being socially gracious were easy, everyone would be kind, courteous and thoughtful all the time, including me. And Miss Manners, Emily Post and Letitia Baldrige would be collecting unemployment alongside other polite, well-mannered folk.

Believe it or not, a decade later, playing bridge with Cyndee has become great fun. It's no surprise that she's a good player and a savvy bidder. But what is a surprise is that she is a much more gracious opponent and partner, which makes it easier for me to admit that she really is a better cardplayer. Equally interesting is this: while the game of bridge requires careful communication and deliberate play, we are no less aware of each other's flaws and habits when it comes to playing the game. Good manners, social graces and the rules of bridge gently ensure that those flaws (mine and hers) don't get in the way of a game well played and enjoyed.

And while good manners and social graces can cure all kinds of societal ills, it's amazing that women who are happy to bask in the glow of their accomplishments—whether bridge, tennis or work—still struggle with graciously accepting a compliment about their appearance. I have heard that we hand out more compliments down south than in more reserved parts of the country, but there should be some universal rules when it comes to giving and receiving compliments with grace—and brevity.

Sure, appearances of effortless beauty can smack a bit of false humility. Likewise, there is the unattractive extreme of showcasing, discussing and dissecting every beauty decision. Women discussing new bolt-on appendages and all-day derm appointments and perpetuating the TMI attitude of "it takes a lot of time and money to look like this . . ." It's as unseemly and inappropriate as discussing money. And besides, it's likely people already know how much money you have, along with how you earned it, if you inherited it, if you're managing it wisely and if you're treating your mother-in-law with generous love and respect. After all, we know you have more money than Croesus and can afford to fly her first-class to Richmond to visit her sister four times a year, what with all that single-barrel, small-batch bourbon you special-order from Kentucky and pretend to give to clients when we all really know you keep it locked in your desk drawer in the library. It's as bad as that.

Accepting a compliment gracefully is simple. At its core it's an appropriately genuine response that acknowledges the compliment and the person paying the compliment. Much like the perfect volley in tennis—you don't lob the ball into the net, nor do you slam it down your opponent's throat.

Exhibit A: "That is a lovely dress you're wearing."

Inappropriate response #1 (delivered with sly satisfaction): "Well, when I saw it, I just had to have it. But the store didn't have it in azure, so my stylist had to call all over the place and finally found it at the Highland Park store in Dallas. Of course, I had to pay to have it FedEx'd so I could wear it to the luncheon at the club. Thank heavens Janine wasn't wearing it, we have showed up TWICE at that luncheon wearing the same dress and I nearly fired my stylist."

Inappropriate response #2 (delivered with an eye roll): "Really, you have to be kidding. I just pulled it out and threw it on."

Appropriate response (delivered with solid eye contact and a smile): "Thank you!"

Exhibit B: "You look great—have you lost weight?"

Inappropriate response #1 (delivered in a conspiratorial tone as you pull up a chair to settle in for the long haul): "Well, you wouldn't believe the amount of money I've paid for the nutritionist, the personal trainer, the supplements, the colonics session—those were a doozy—the gym and spa membership and the workout gear. Jeez, I could have gone to a fat farm in the south of France for a month! Do you know what else? My tennis partner pretended not to notice how much my serve had improved since I started all this stuff. As if."

Inappropriate response #2 (delivered with eyes wide with false wonder): "I just don't understand it, but when I'm stressed, the weight just falls off."

Appropriate response (delivered with solid eye contact and a smile): "I *have* lost weight! I've been working hard, so thanks for noticing."

Just like sleep begets sleep, accepting compliments graciously tends to generate more of them. And like my socially astute sisters, I have to practice like the best of them. The graceful formula: eye contact, plus a smile, and a genuine "thank you!"—

is a hard habit to form and to deliver. So I was pleased as punch when I realized my teen daughter had perfected her response to a compliment. Her "thank you" manages to sound equal parts delighted that you noticed, appreciative that you said something at all and genuinely grateful for the kind words. As if your offering up of a compliment was a dash of sprinkles on what was already the cupcake of the day—a lovely little finish.

Never had the need for a lovely little finish been more apparent than when I came to grips with the DMV. I was running errands one winter afternoon a few years ago, racking up minutes on my iPhone by gabbing with my girlfriend and neighbor. Between stops at the bank, the dry cleaner and the grocery store, we were swapping supposed shortcomings—poor time management, feeding our kids pigs-in-a-blanket for dinner (her, not me, for the record), not washing our face every night before bed (that was totally me, but I'm just so beat) and so on. It evolved into one of those silly chats where we were trying to top each other with appalling (not really) admissions of bad parenting (a bit possible), bad grooming (totally possible) or bad spousal relations (not at ALL possible; remember, I am the girl who did the deed with my husband for an ENTIRE YEAR).

"I have an expired driver's license," I admitted. "I haven't really told anyone. I'm not sure Brad knows." My admission was both a confession and an attempt to top my pal's recent litany of transgressions.

"Oh puleeze. That's not that bad. How long has it been expired?"

"More than two years." There was a long pause on the phone.

"Two years? Are you kidding? That's unreal," she said. I couldn't discern if it was awe or judgment that I heard in her voice. "I can't believe you haven't been pulled over," she continued. "If you do, I have a great lawyer, by the way," my friend said as I took the corner of Runnymede Lane on two wheels.

"I know, it's bad. But I am a very good driver," I said with a grin as I wrapped up our conversation and mentally committed to get on the monumental task of renewing my driver's license.

In addition to being a very good driver, I am a very alert driver. Speeding tickets? Not since college. Expired registration? Not since college. Expired license plates? Not since college. Expired license? Not since I turned forty and could not find EIGHT uninterrupted hours to drive myself to the DMV and get a new license. Since then, all air travel required my passport (and birth certificate . . . and marriage certificate), which is a slight hassle. And I was always a bit worried that the bank would decline to cash a check. So the hassle of living life with an expired license outweighed the hassle of spending an entire day in line at the DMV with the rest of the world. I mean, it's one thing to spend the day at the park (open to the general public) or the mall (certainly open to the general public), but the DMV? No thank you, ma'am.

But the day of reckoning had come. I couldn't wait any longer—quite honestly, living outside the law in such a reckless and wanton manner was simply too much for this nerdy girl. And since you probably don't know what happens when you show up at the DMV with a license that's been expired for more than two years, because you're simply not that slack (or lazy), I'll tell you.

Before you leave the house, you find your birth certificate, your marriage license, your passport, a utility bill that documents your address, a compass, a small, soft cooler of Diet Cokes, a flare gun and a notarized copy of your last will and testament. After all, who knows when you'll be back, right? And you make sure that you're dressed in a snappy, business-casual outfit that shows you care. And then you get in a really, really *nice* frame of mind. Because this is a day when my dad's adage of "Be nice to everyone" rings true.

What he didn't say was "Be nice, sweet daughter, because you might be kissing some major DMV booty as you try to sweet-talk your way into an updated license that doesn't have a photo of you sporting fourteen chins. And by the way, what in the world were you thinking to let your license expire like that?" Or that's what my dad might say if he knew. Luckily he didn't, so I could drive to the DMV in peace, at the crack of dawn, in a perky and brightly colored twin sweater set and some nice sling-back wedges, in the lame hope that I might be first in line. Which never, ever happens because there are always people waiting in line at the DMV, no matter what the time of day. Even on holidays. Even at night. Even when the DMV is closed, there are still people waiting in line, no? I predict that when the world comes to an end, people will be running around in mass hysteria and apocalyptic panic, and still there will be people, you guessed it, standing in line at the DMV.

To continue, once you arrive at the office, you are immediately triaged, just like in the ER. Paperwork in check? Go to that desk. New citizen and first-time license? No chance, friend, head on home and wait for a better day.

And if you're me, you find you're missing a very important insurance document. So you call your insurance agent (thank goodness my aunt Karen answered) in a panic and beg her to fax Form E#12583482373543449587348957234895 7438754 posthaste to the wide, bored, good-ol'-boy DMV officer sitting at a special desk in a roped-off area (yes, as if he's KING of the DMV). Because out of the reams of paperwork I bring to the DMV to document my birth, my marriage, my citizenship, my home state and where I want my children to reside in the case of my untimely death, I didn't bring Form E#12583482373543 49587348957234895 7438754. That's why it's smart to have a family member or longtime family friend as a service provider (insurance, doctor, plumber). Immediate access is key.

Once good-ol'-boy DMV officer received proof that I owned and drove an insured vehicle, I took a number (like at the deli), took a load off and a look around. I was sitting in a linoleum-lined, fluorescent-lighted nearly windowless box where dreams of a beautiful near future go to die, I was sure of it.

I sat between a woman with a newborn baby and another woman in a floor-length burka, with my paperwork laying unattended in my lap. I was riveted.

Why would a brand-new mom with a brand-new baby be at the DMV . . . by herself . . . in a germy, gross, smelly office with lots of strangers? I knew that I had nipped MRSA in the bud and had taken a shower this morning, but I could only vouch for myself, and all these people were cooing and fussing over this tiny little baby. I mean, if you want to show off your baby, can't you go to the park? Or to the grocery store? And I can assure you that getting a license photo taken days after giving birth is not going to happen in my lifetime. Don't new moms get some kind of temporary DMV exemption? Can't they have one of those shadow heads in the photo?

Next, I turned to the woman in the floor-length, face-covering burka. Where to begin? Does she have to show her face in her license photo? Can she drive with her face covered? Is that fair? Is that legal? Is that attractive? Is that a good idea for me?

The DMV is a petri dish of humanity and I couldn't seem to turn away. It's not every day (or even every decade, come to think of it) that I visit the DMV. I'm like a drunk at the ABC store, I can't drink it in fast enough.

They finally called my number, and I was seated in front of a senior-level, official-looking DMV officer who started furiously typing and interrogating me. Officer Carr was an older, neatly groomed black man with a nicely trimmed mustache, graying sideburns, wire-rimmed glasses and an orderly desk. As he was inputting my information, he shared the ever-so-important, oh-so-tiny tidbit of news that in addition to taking the written driving exam, I had to take the road test.

I nearly choked on my Diet Coke. "Um, excuse me, Officer

Carr. Could you repeat that? I thought I heard you say that I would have to take an exam AND the road test?" I was looking down at my unopened test booklet that was buried in my paperwork.

"That's right, Mrs. Muller," Officer Carr replied, peering over his glasses with a look so bored and so done with me he might as well have said, "I am so over you little Junior League moms thinking they can float on over here to Albemarle Road when the mood hits and float right out of here with a shiny new license." He didn't say it out loud, of course, but he might as well have.

What he did say was: "All persons with a license expired more than one year are required to take the road test. And it appears your license has been expired for over two years. Is that right, Mrs. Muller?" Again, I got that over-the-glasses stink eye.

"Um, yes, that's right. But, Officer Carr, I don't think I've taken a road test since, well"—I was doing some quick math in my head, not my strong suit—"since 1983. Do they still have the driver's cars with brakes on the passenger's side?" I was trying to offer some levity and to reinforce the fact that I was FORTY-FREAKIN'-TWO YEARS OLD!

"Mrs. Muller, I don't know where you took your road test. But I think you're referring to a Driver Education Vehicle. You are required to take the driving test in your own vehicle. You do have a licensed and insured vehicle on property?"

Huh? That set off a whole other set of worries—I mean, I did have a licensed and insured vehicle on property (just ask good-ol'-boy DMV officer five desks down). But did I even have any gas? How many crushed Diet Coke cans and Chick-fil-A wrappers would come falling out when he opened the door to climb in my filthy SUV? Did my car still smell like fermented chocolate milk? Was I going to have to parallel park? If I failed, would someone have to come get me? I mean, you couldn't really LEAVE the DMV without a valid license and get in a car and just drive away, could you? Didn't they have spotters or something?

So Officer Carr typed away, asking questions, confirming facts. I answered promptly, with lots of "yes sirs" and "no sirs." I was very nice. I worked to appear contrite. Which, at this point, was easy. I was woefully and sincerely and unbelievably contrite. I couldn't believe I had let this happen. I was far too old to be sitting here, hat in hand, with an expired license, at the mercy of the North Carolina Division of Motor Vehicles and Officer Carr.

"Mrs. Muller, I'm going to ask you to step over to the exam area for the written test. You will be taking the test in English, correct?"

"What are my options?" I asked, trying again for a bit of levity. I don't know why I was bent on getting Officer Carr to like me . . . even just a *little* bit. But the man couldn't be broken, despite all my polite charm and earnest manners.

"I repeat, English or Spanish. Are you bilingual, Mrs. Muller? Would you prefer to take the test in Spanish?"

"No, sir," I replied, "I'm not bilingual. English is just fine." I looked down at a chewed thumbnail. All of a sudden my cute sweater set didn't seem so bright and cheery.

"There are twenty-five questions on the test. To pass, you

must score an eighty or better. Do you know how many questions you must get correct, Mrs. Muller?"

I turned the slow turbine of my math brain over. "I need to get twenty questions correct to pass, Officer Carr," I responded.

"Very good, Mrs. Muller." He acted genuinely impressed. "Are you a schoolteacher?" he asked, looking over his glasses at me.

"No, sir. I just had some good ones. But an eighty? That seems kinda high. What happened to the seventy as a standard passing grade?"

"Twenty out of twenty-five questions, Mrs. Muller. I hope you studied. If you fail, you can take the test again. But you should know, there are five tests that rotate randomly in the computers. You can't study to the test, as you'll never know which test you'll get. It's better to have studied all the material." Ah, at least some government hack somewhere had caught on to the strategy of teaching to the test.

Okay, folks, it's not going to give away the ending when I tell you that I didn't study ANY OF THE MATERIAL. And we don't need to get into all the reasons why, the least of which is that I was dumb enough to assume that since I'd been driving for TWENTY-SIX YEARS I knew all I needed to know about U-turns, merge lanes and parallel parking. And, for a middle-aged gal with ADD, the DMV waiting area is like crack. Besides, that woman in the burka was taking her test, and I was dying to know if she passed.

So after running through different doomsday scenarios, one of which included the actual execution of my last will and testament, I was seized with a burst of the obvious. There were some pretty thick people driving cars, trucks and Harleys in the state of North Carolina, and they managed to pass the test. How hard could it be? If some lactating mother with raging hormones running on no sleep could pass this test, surely I could, too. I worked to get in a DMV zone. Focused . . . calm . . . logical (all things NOT DMV). I breathed in deeply and started to think about my daughter's test-taking strategy—take your time, read all the questions thoroughly, rule out the obvious, answer the questions you know and then come back to the ones you don't.

I sat down, put on my earphones and started cranking through the test. Here is the weird thing. You know RIGHT THEN if you answered the question correctly and the system doesn't allow you to skip ahead. This saves everyone time. So if you miss the first six questions, there's really no need to answer the last nineteen—you've already flunked and they send you away to hitch a ride home. Likewise, if you don't miss one question, you only end up answering twenty questions instead of twenty-five—you've passed with the requisite twenty correct answers, so why worry about a higher score? Apparently, the DMV settles for chronic mediocrity—everyone makes an eighty—OR NOT. That says a lot, don't you think?

I scored my eighty with one question remaining. Whew. Mediocrity ruled.

I would like to publicly state that every question I missed related to drinking and driving—how much time I would serve if convicted of drunk driving, how much time I would serve if I bought alcohol for an underage driver, how much would I pay in court costs/fines if I was pulled over for drunk driving, etc. It never occurred to me to know that stuff because I've never been *that* driver. But it also seemed banal: does the DMV think people AREN'T going to do these things because they studied for and learned about the horrible legal ramifications of drunk driving on their DMV test? By the way, any questions that had to do with, say, *actual driving*? I aced those, as I am a very good driver.

Relief flooded through me. This whole drama had taken more energy than I'd imagined. I headed back to Officer Carr's desk, ready for my next assignment. I felt like I was applying for college—the essay, the standardized tests, interviews with admissions. My cute outfit was now a bit crumpled. The ice was melting in my little cooler. The woman in the burka was long gone—her fate unknown to me. I had lost all sense of time and space in this DMV vortex. Officer Carr looked at me.

"Congratulations, Mrs. Muller, you passed the written portion of the test."

"Thank you, Officer Carr. It was touch and go there for a while." I was not kidding this time. Even so, I thought I saw a little, ever-so-slight pull at the corner of his mouth.

"Mrs. Muller, it is within a DMV officer's consideration to waive the need for a road test if he or she thinks it appropriate."

I looked closely at Officer Carr, nervously trying to iron out the wrinkles in my khaki pants with my hands, then straightened up and looked him in the eye. I couldn't tell if he was yanking my chain or throwing me a line but I took the bait.

"Officer Carr, I am hoping that today might be my lucky day

and that you might consider it appropriate to waive my road test." I was trying to be nice—really very nice, and genuinely respectful and appropriately contrite. All things my parents beat into me at a very early age, along with "Pretty is as pretty does" and "Always keep your gas tank more than half full."

"Indeed it is, Mrs. Muller, your lucky day, courtesy of the North Carolina Division of Motor Vehicles. It seems you have an outstanding driving record, despite your lapsed license," he said, finally cracking a just barely perceptible smile.

"Officer Carr, I cannot thank you enough," I said. With that, I gathered up my reams of paperwork and my cooler, wrote my thirty-five-dollar check and bounced over to the "picture" station, where I sang out "Cheese!" to the camera. Joy overflowed in my DMV photo, I must say. Being nice helps you get places, including HOME from the DMV with a newly minted driver's license in hand, not set to expire for another six years.

I have spent the last four years of that six-year DMV exemption wisely by driving safely (most of the time), obeying all traffic signals (some of the time) and working to teach my kids social graces and manners (most all of the time). And because we're in the South, that includes cotillion. Cotillions historically were designed to prepare debutantes for their coming-out parties. But by all modern definitions, cotillion is a series of classes that offer instruction in dancing, manners, deportment, and other social graces (like excusing oneself to a private place to discharge gas, and trimming one's nails in private and over a sink). For me, cotillion was a form of seventh-grade hell, made even more hellish when I finally got to dance (up close) with the boy of my dreams (one Jack Johnson) only to realize that I, alas, had more facial hair and height than he did. I was not, at the time, the socially skilled individual that I am today and it was a disaster.

Unlike me, my daughter breezed through her own cotillion classes, which were filled with happy, well-groomed friends she had known since kindergarten. And no one smelled. She seemed fairly unaffected and actually enjoyed it.

"Mom, do you know what Mrs. Perkins said you are supposed to do if you're at a party and not having a good time?" she asked the morning after one of her cotillion classes.

I threw out a few options. Hide in the bathroom and cry in the handicapped stall? Stage a protest, take hostages and demand social equity for all? Set something on fire?

"Fake it!" she announced with a gleeful grin on her face. "Mrs. Perkins said that if you pretend you are having a good time when you're not, you just might end up having a good time anyway."

I stopped everything I was doing and turned to face her. The etiquette skies had opened and politely dropped a beautifully wrapped gift into my lap. I was totally writing a thank-you note (on my really nice monogrammed stationery) for this one.

"Mrs. Perkins was absolutely right," I said. "Sometimes you just need to fake it and pretend you are having a good time. And sometimes you just might." I looked my daughter straight in the eyes. "Please don't EVER forget those words. If I can leave this world knowing I imparted a few nuggets of insight that I plagiarized from your cotillion teacher, I will consider myself an incredible mom." And I still believe that to be true. Even middle age and seasoned social acumen don't preempt the need to some-times pretend you're having a good time when you're not. And the same can be said of getting pretty—*acting* pretty is half the battle, and that requires some good manners and a nice dose of social graces (and an elegant glass of your favorite Pinot in your right hand always helps, too).

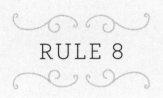

RULE 8

The Mirror Doesn't Lie and Neither Does Your Mother

My friend Ruth and I were shopping at a lovely little women's boutique in our hometown of Asheville, a funky, artsy city where college students roam alongside retirees at great restaurants, breweries and galleries. We were visiting on a girls' bridge weekend and a group of us were buzzing around a charming shopping village in twos and threes. As we knocked around the small, intimate ladies' boutique that took up four small rooms in a historic bungalow, we came across a mother and her teen daughter. The teen was trying on frock after frock, looking for what would be the "perfect" dress to wear to a Mother-Daughter Symphony Tea.

NEWSFLASH: For a fourteen-year-old, the perfect dress doesn't exist. No dress has the magical power to transform you into something you're not. This is not intended to be harsh, but rather a universal acknowledgment of the unrealistic dreams we all had as awkward teenagers. And if you lived an unabashedly

UN-awkward life as a teenager and none of this resonates with you, then just skip ahead.

The daughter was lovely, with a small waist and strong, athletic legs. She was trying on dresses that were oh-so-in-style—short, satiny, boxlike and bright. Think poly-Puccis. But what was the style du jour for über-conscious tweens did nothing to showcase her specific features. The mother and the sales associate guided the daughter toward more flattering dresses—longer, with cinched waists and pretty necklines that drew the eye to the face. Much like my mother steered me away from pleated waistlines and formfitting tops.

But the daughter was no fool—she knew that the more flattering dresses for her were the less trendy ones. The mother was whispering loudly in the dressing room, pointing to (I imagine) the dresses she was willing to purchase and those that were absolutely "out of the question and not appropriate." The daughter settled into a borderline whine, ticking off every OTHER girl she knew who would attend wearing something incredibly fashion-forward. There was a younger sister, bored out of her mind and sprawled out in an upholstered chair outside the dressing room, with her nose in a book.

The unflappable sales associate was clicking through the racks looking for more options. I assumed this was old hat to her—the delicate balancing act between mothers and daughters, between what flatters and what does not, between what the mother would finance and what the daughter would deign to wear. My insides churned at the familiarity of it all. The teen angst of fitting in when, really, things didn't fit that well to begin with. The maternal angst of helping your daughter present well without having to break the news that she will NEVER be shaped like [fill in the blank]. Are mothers wrong and misguided in their attempts to strong-arm fashion? Perhaps. Are teenage daughters petulant and all-knowing as they pose for a photo that they will one day burn in utter humiliation? Of course.

But I will tell you this—my mother was right more times than she was wrong. And I'm willing to take those odds with my daughter. Because at the end of the day, there is one fashion truth: your mother really does want what is best for you . . . because what is best for you often is what is best for her. Translation: when you look good, she looks good.

Boom. Done. End of story.

Mothers have a way of telling it like it is. I was twelve when my mother and I pulled up outside a friend's house. As I opened the car door to get out, my mom beckoned me to stay put. She would only be a minute. I protested—I wanted to go in and visit with my friend. We got into a spat that ended only when my mother announced that my hair looked like it had been parked in cooking oil, that my body odor was so overwhelming that she could barely breathe and that there was no way I was going inside that house in my current state.

Well, talk about hitting a prepubescent, oily-faced, husky-size preteen when she's down.

Wanna dose of real life? Go shopping with your mother. Because those three-way mirrors with the fluorescent lights don't lie. And neither does your mother. I never ask my husband if an outfit makes me look frumpy, dumpy. Not because I don't care, because I really, really do care. It's that I don't trust his answer. Want to know if your butt looks big in those Seven jeans? Ask your mom or your girlfriend. Women don't dress for men, they dress for other women. Except for those women who wear skimpy tank tops that reveal harrowing amounts of cleavage—no, those women are dressing for men. But everyone else? We're constantly appraising each other—hair, makeup, shoes, complexion, neck wattle, you name it.

Now I have become my mother.

I admit it: how my kids look and dress (and of course, smell) is a reflection, for better or for worse, on me. I expect them to look halfway decent for a piano recital or church, and I feel sure I'm not denying "who they are" or squashing their individuality when I ask one to wear a sport coat and tie, and the other a nice dress. If I am pushing some standards and expectations on them, well, is that wrong? Consider it a public service. I think we feel our ability to contribute to the world often rides on the perfect complexion of our offspring. Darwin knew it then and women know it now. Pretty gets you far(ther).

All told, most of us like our mothers. Sure, there are women who hate their mothers. Perhaps their mothers were narcissistic, selfish, self-absorbed creatures who never should have spawned another human—but those gals are few and far between and we can usually spot them (and run the other way). They're drug-addled actresses floating in and out of rehab. They're the PTA president who takes no prisoners when it comes to making sure you do your time in the volunteer gulag. There's the opposite side of the spectrum as well—friends whose mothers rank right up there with Mary Poppins and Maria von Trapp. The rest of us fall in between—we love our moms, we fight with them, we ignore them, they ignore us (at least we think they do, and how dare they!), we let them tell us things about our children that no other human would be allowed to utter without a fight. And we let them tell us when we look really, really crappy in something. Because remember, when we look good, they look good.

In many ways, it's obvious that all our "stuff" about looks, appearances and beauty comes from our mothers. The majority of our opinions on beauty and aging and appearances and the frequency of waxing most likely come from our moms. They set us straight in many cases, and let's face it, screwed us up. The only reason I can say this with a fair amount of authority is that I'm doing it now to my own daughter. For better or for worse, mothers and daughters and beauty and worth are all tangled up like a giant round roller brush. To separate mothers and daughters from beauty, appearance and the life lessons learned in PE classes is like separating water from rain. You can't do it without changing the very essence of one or the other.

In fact, I suggest that one can't really survive without the other—that sort of twisted and disturbing parasitic relationship that your therapist warns you about.

I am a spooky reflection of my mother—and of her mother—dark, hooded eyes, heavy eyebrows and a dimple, barely noticeable, at the corner of the mouth when we smile. A dimple now lightly embedded in the delicate face of my niece.

Recently, I asked my mother if I could borrow her mink coat to wear to an evening event. It was a black-tie social event and we were attending with a few couples. I trust that what looks great on her will work on me. I also figured it would be campy and fab, and über warm, as it weighs as much as a small infant. And now that my mother is a snowbird and leaves her mountain town during the winter for the warmth and comfort of the Florida coast, she hardly wears the coat.

"Hey, Mom, you know that awesome black-tie party Brad and I are planning to attend?" I threw out one afternoon when we were chatting on the phone. "I thought perhaps I could please borrow your mink coat for the event?"

"Um, I don't know, sweetie." Huge pause here. "You might lose it."

Lose a fourteen-pound fur coat? Is she kidding? What am I—TWELVE? And then I realized that, on some level, to her, perhaps I am. Even though we're both grown up now, I'm in my forties and she's in her sixties, maybe she doesn't see me as grown up enough yet to have earned the right to wear her full-length mink coat that she received as an anniversary gift from my father and that has a careful hand monogram (HER monogram, by the way, not mine) on the inside silk lining. That despite how much we have in common, how much we look alike and how much we share, there is some kind of hierarchy to the sharing. Because we are not peers. Just because I *could* wear my mother's three-inch pumps when I was twelve didn't mean I *should* wear my mother's three-inch pumps. She rightly said no then. And she rightly said no again. (But, girlfriend, it would've looked F-A-B, I do know that much.)

Once Mom hit Florida, I believe it took her about 8.6 seconds to sniff out the Jewish jewelry mall. And she didn't even have her mink coat to use as a homing device.

The bastion of all things that glitter and sparkle, the Jewish jewelry mall sits in a strip shopping center a few blocks off the Interstate 95 interchange. Behind display cabinets overflowing with diamonds, gold, platinum and stones stood men in yarmulkes and women with perfectly manicured fingers clad in double-digit carats. It's as if a tornado picked up a block of stores from Manhattan's diamond district and plopped it on the I-95 off-ramp. Bells tinkled when my mother and I entered. Eager eyes spotted us and the dance began.

"Let me know if there is anything I can help with," offered up one salesperson at the counter on our right.

"That's a gor-jus medallion. Come closer—let me look," commented another, this one to our left.

And then the mother of all enticements: "Are you and your sister looking for anything special?"

That one stopped my mother and me both in our tracks. We both looked at the salesclerk at yet a different counter—she was dressed in slacks and a blouse, with an efficient and appropriate hairstyle. She peered at us over her glasses and waited. My mother broke the spell with a light laugh and a sheepish smile.

"Oh my, this is my DAUGHTER," she said with exaggerated emphasis.

The salesclerk looked back and forth between the two of us. I looked at her with a raised brow in silent confirmation. Then the clerk started tittering about how great we both looked and how our features were so similar that we could be twins and blah, blah, blah and wasn't it all just a hoot? I strolled down the center aisle away from the salesclerk and my mother, trailed my fingers along the glass and pretended to gaze at all the pretties. I threw over my shoulder with a droll shrug, "Just remember, it's only a compliment to one of us."

But the saleslady in the jewelry store played it well—accidental or not, she had complimented the "sister" with the generous jewelry budget. They put their heads together like two little hens and pecked their way through trays and trays of pretty bracelets. I turned and looked at my reflection in a mirror and searched for the signs that connected my mother and me as sisters.

My mother's appearance used to forecast mine—what I might look like at twenty, thirty or forty.

As I get older and she works to stay younger, it's like some sort of trippy time travel. Now we're compared by strangers to sisters. The mother (with some excellent work) and the daughter (clearly in need of some) have met in the middle of their twenty-four-year age divide. Now we come across as pretty peers. The comment brought my mother joy, perhaps some satisfaction; how could it not? I'm not sure what it brought me. As an only daughter, I don't have competing beauty interests and, by the same token, beauty colleagues. There's no one with whom I can compare notes on who received the most "pretty perks."

My sister-in-law Elise has two beautiful sisters. Their mother is lovely, and they all drank from the same gorgeous gene pool. "But Maria was always the prettiest," Elise would comment about her oldest sister. "And as pretty as my mother is, she had sisters whom she considered prettier." The generosity of sisters amazes me—I cannot find one who is not willing to pass the pretty title to another, as if it is some unwritten code. No one ever insisted I was prettier and now I'm in ever-so-subtle competition with the first person to ever announce my pretty—my mother. It is vexing.

My friend Kate is not allowed this luxury of up-close-and-personal maternal beauty introspection. Her mother died a year after Kate married, a victim of early-onset Alzheimer's. But Kate does look like her mother—remarkably so—the deep-set, almond-shaped eyes; the petite, pear-shaped figure; pretty bow-shaped lips and the narrow face with the camera-ready jawline. Sitting on a handsome sideboard in her roomy kitchen is a picture of Kitty, Kate's mother and namesake, a candid black-and-white photo from the early seventies. Her hair is pulled away from her face in an effortless and appropriate bouffantlike do, her face is bright and relaxed, wearing a half smile and pale pink frosty lipstick. She is lovely. If Kate can't look into the mirror of her mother's face, she can look at that photo and see the transitive property of familial beauty. If A=B and B=C, then A=C. If Kate's mother is beautiful and Kate looks like her mother, then Kate must be beautiful, too. It is true: she is.

Charla Muller

Will my daughter be able to do that? After all is said and done, will I overcorrect my perceived flaws to a point where my daughter cannot reflect in my image, nor I in hers? In an effort to emulate my daughter's youth, will I erase the very things that connect us? I'm not sure I have the restraint, but while I've dabbled in Botox, stood naked (nearly) as a jaybird for a bronzed spray tan and wholly embraced Lasik eye surgery, I've not done anything (yet) that I can't take back. I don't even have a tattoo lurking somewhere discreet, waiting in the wings to prove that I am indeed a cool, hip forty-something mom (which I'm so not).

When my daughter was younger, there was tangible and concrete value in the things that connected us—bake from scratch her favorite cookies, coordinate a favorite playdate, present well during Parents' Night at school. It was a real kick to watch her age and mature and with that age and maturity come to realize that there are less tangible but possibly more valuable things that I might bring to the table.

"Mom, do you know how Sarah and her mom look so much alike? They both have freckles and the same color hair?" my daughter asked one day while the two of us were driving to her brother's baseball game. She was around ten and it was an away game that required a forty-five-minute cross-county commute. It was spring and there was still a bite of chill in the air.

"Mm-hmm," I responded as I merged carefully onto the interstate, glancing at my rearview mirror.

"Well, you and I are alike, too," she said, staring out the window. "We're both funny and creative and can write really good stories. And we can make our friends laugh." Well, I'll be.

If I could have pulled over right then on the side of Interstate 85, hopped out of my gas-guzzling (but very safe) SUV and dropped to my knees in thanks to the good Lord who instilled in that sweet thing something that people pay THOUSANDS of dollars for in therapy, I would have done it. Because I know that one day she will yell at me and blame me and curse me for the flabby elbows and "poochy tummy" she inherited from me (and I won't blame her). But I'm so thankful she can see that I'm bringing more to the table than scratch-baked cookies and a unibrow. That on some level she knows and understands that while she will inherit and likely need to cultivate some pretty qualities (like her thick gorgeous hair), she will also inherit and likely need to cultivate some qualities that make her interesting (like her witty personality). And just like our definition of pretty should grow and evolve as we grow (older) and (more) evolved, so should how we define it to others, much like my daughter did.

"Hon," I announced one November night from the dining room. My desk had spread like the Blob, slowly oozing and creeping into the adjoining room. "If there comes a day when you can't find me, and I mean that literally, look for me under a pile of paperwork."

I'm not talking about work paperwork; I'm talking about kid paperwork. There is not one aspect of my children's lives that is not documented by unceasing paperwork—transportation, sports, photo releases, back to school, end of school, band, church, choir, fall sports, spring sports, camp, you name it. So when I got an update from the sixth-grade band instructor, I put it in a to-do pile that sits higher than my dirty laundry (and that's saying something). I got to it when . . . well, when I got to it.

"Did you know that we are REQUIRED to attend the middle school holiday band performance?" I called out to my husband.

"Well, wouldn't we go anyway?" he shouted over his shoulder as he lounged on the sofa and watched football. My husband has a soft spot for band concerts, as he was a band geek on steroids.

"Probably," I replied. "But I just don't like to be TOLD I HAVE to go to a sixth-grade band concert."

I kept going. "What if I was some famous heart surgeon who was called in to perform delicate surgery on some international diplomat who is in the U.S. as part of sensitive negotiations that could impact world peace as we know it, and I simply couldn't attend the mandatory middle school band concert?"

"I guess it's a good thing you aren't," said my husband, O he of the wit as dry as burned toast.

You know WHY the sixth-grade band teacher required parents to attend? Because if she didn't, parents everywhere (including famous cardiac surgeons) would screech into the parking lot on two wheels, open the door and spit out a tuba and a penguin (a kid in black pants and a white shirt) and head down to the local bowling alley for free wings and pitchers of beer. Because parents were once kids and we all know this to be true: stay away from the band concert.

"Oh, and get a load of this!" I barked, even more worked up. "This *mandatory* band concert is the first Friday night in December." It was September.

"What, do you already have plans?" he volleyed back.

"Well, I PLAN to have plans," I crisply retorted

I was annoyed. The first Friday in December is valuable real estate when it comes to parties, drop-ins, Book Club celebration, neighborhood ornament swaps, gingerbread-house-decorating parties, caroling outings and any other fa-la-la events. I had every intention of being triple-booked and simply unable to attend the mandatory band concert. I mean, what was this band director thinking?

It didn't matter what she was thinking, as all of my band-o-phobic ranting and raving was met with the ultimate in karmic payback—I didn't receive a SINGLE invitation to attend some swank (or otherwise) holiday soiree the first Friday in December. It appeared that I had all the time in the world to attend the MANDATORY middle school band concert. And so I did.

My mother, who was in town that weekend, attended, too. She was gearing up for her annual migration to Florida in a few weeks and wanted to bond with the grandkids before she flew the coop.

When heading south, my mother has two goals: the first is to pack every single item one might need to survive a nuclear holocaust. The second is to arrive healthy and well. Because once in Florida, she will be basking in large amounts of vitamin D, playing bridge, painting and attending cocktail parties every evening at six sharp.

As such, attending a December band concert in a dank, underground cement space with lots of adults and children had Mom worried. So she did what anyone would do. She showed up in a full-length mink coat and a surgical mask.

"Mom, are you serious? You're wearing a surgical mask!"

"Who knows what kinds of germs lurk in a middle school auditorium? Besides, you can't really see it if I wrap this pretty pashmina around my face like so."

No, you couldn't see the face mask, as my mother looked like a member of the cashmere al-Qaeda.

"Don't worry, I'll stand in the back," she offered as we parked and hustled into the building.

The school auditorium sits in the bowels of a decades-old building that smells like every other school auditorium in the free world. If smells were emotions, they would be odors of angst, restlessness and possibility. Deeply familiar.

In an effort to salvage that Friday night in December, I tried to rally a few families to go to dinner after the concert. But I misjudged the length of this wonderful musicale. Apparently, not only were we required to attend a band concert on one of the most important holiday evenings of the year, but we were also required to stay the entire time. I couldn't skip out after the sixth-grade portion of the evening. I had to sit through the seventh- and eighth-grade concerts, too.

Finally, it was the changing of the bands. Penguins of all shapes and sizes flooded the stage while a different tribe of penguins stared out into the abyss of creaky auditorium seats looking for their parents. Our daughter settled in next to me. As some kid with a French horn squeezed past us, I patted her knee and pointed out that her grandmother was the short gal in the back dressed like an upscale terrorist.

In the meantime, I was trying to text my pal Cyndee, who had arrived early and was sitting up front (because apparently it's a crush for the good seats at those mandatory middle school band concerts). My text was not going through. After several tries, I realized the problem—cinderblock walls, our underground location.

So I did what anyone would do. I raised my iPhone in the air as far as my short, stubby arm would allow, hoping that another thirty-six inches would make all the difference.

"Mom!" my daughter hissed. I mean it, she hissed at me, like a black-and-white iguana. "What are you doing?"

"My text to Cyndee isn't going through. I think it's because we're in this underground bunker." I turned to her with my arm still in the air. "I think this will help."

"Would you please stop that?" she said, again with the hiss. "You are embarrassing me!"

A look of disbelief spread across my face. My daughter was slumped down in her seat, trying to disappear behind her flute. The girl is thin, but not that thin. I could tell she was tempted to grab that guy's French horn, too. I bit my tongue, lowered my arm and prayed for a modicum of patience.

What I was dying to say that evening, but I didn't, was a truth that mothers everywhere want to scream to their young at painful moments like middle school band concerts.

"You're kidding, right? I can't possibly be embarrassing

you because EVERYTHING about this entire evening is embar-
rassing! We're at a middle school band concert. You have a
grandmother posing as a terrorist. A younger brother slumped
at the end of the row, asleep. Your mother is in a foul mood
because she didn't get invited to ONE holiday function and now
she seriously regrets that she didn't make a run at medical
school, as she could be operating on some foreign dignitary at
this VERY MOMENT! And now she can't find anyone who
wants to go out for ice cream."

And while I was right, I didn't say it. There will be other times
when I will need to speak the truth, but this wasn't one of them.
Like mothers before me, I bit my tongue, pasted on a smile, lowered my arm and settled in for hour two of the middle school
band concert. Later, I sorted through all the strange elements of
the evening and reflected on my often awkward, clunky childhood and the number of times my mother must have bitten her
tongue. For as many times as she spoke truth, there had to have
been twice as many times when she held back—saving the truth
for another day, or deciding it was a truth that wasn't all that
important, or perhaps she was simply at a loss for how to speak it.

Because mothers know, and while they might not offer up their
wide-open opinion every time the opportunity presents itself,
they don't lie. And we often know it, too, don't we? Like our
daughters, we see it in the flicker of emotion that flashes across
their faces. We hear it in the words not spoken. We experience
it by way of an afternoon of shopping. We daughters spend more

time than we should on the couch in the therapist's office obsessing about our mothers' blunt opinions of us. But at the core, it's a fundamental truth that never changes. We are a reflection of our mothers—both for better and for worse. Most mothers want us to be happy, well-adjusted and well-groomed contributing members of society on the inside and out.

Why? Because they love of us. Boom. Done. End of story.

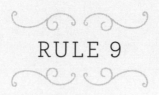

RULE 9

Dress the Part

Remember that spring when Oscar de la Renta and I were chatting in his suite at the Ritz-Carlton? Okay, I wasn't really chatting with Oscar. Rather I was eavesdropping shamelessly on his conversation with a reporter and obnoxiously inserting myself in said conversation because, helloooooo, it was OSCAR DE LA RENTA.

Anyway, Oscar and the reporter were discussing the royal wedding, which had been telecast that day throughout the galaxy, and, of course, they were talking about Kate's dress.

In his fabulously thick, sexy Latin accent, Oscar said, "I loved de drez. It was vury aprupriat to cova de showderz. Today, too menny brides just valk down de aisle and they just geev it all away." There were some accompanying hand gestures to drive the "give it all away" point home.

You heard me right. Oscar de la Renta reinforced the concept of *less is more*. I—the woman who loves cardigans—very nearly wept. But not in front of Oscar, of course. I would muss my makeup.

Folks in my neck of the woods often get accused of sins of excess—big weddings (check); big hair (check); big college football schools (check) and big egos (check). But when it comes to appearance and presentation, you might be surprised to know that many of us have been schooled in the art of restraint and discretion. Less is more. Not every physical feature was meant to be showcased, maximized, teased, enhanced or inflated. And Kate was the poster child for all things appropriate.

Kate Middleton was dressing for the part she was becoming—a princess. Tasteful, demure, appropriate. Nope, Kate wasn't going to waltz down that aisle in a tight, strapless mermaid dress tricked out in sequins and Swarovski crystals. And her dress didn't come in "parts" so she could whip off the bottom half for her bump-and-grind sessions with the groomsmen at the reception. Her dress was an homage to tradition, modesty and discernment as well as a nod to the indisputable fact that the most eligible bachelor in the land had chosen her. For some, it was a walk down memory lane—viewing the royal wedding made them nostalgic for their own wedding and they saw their younger, more innocent selves. Not me.

Back in the late nineties, when it was FINALLY my time to shop for a bridal gown, I wasn't living out one of those over-the-top wedding-dress reality shows or tricking myself out as possible royalty. It was hard work to find a wedding dress that I liked, that played to my figure and that met my mother's exacting standards. Because, remember—when I look good, she looks good and this was her debut role as Mother of the Bride.

And similarly, I saw myself in her image. I was convinced that I would NEVER look as pretty as my mother did in her wedding dress. Growing up, I would spend hours going through the family photo albums stacked in a neat row on the bottom shelf in our den right alongside college and high school yearbooks. Instead of reading classic children's stories and traditional fairy tales, I would spend hours curled up on the floor, thumbing through those albums and yearbooks, creating my own fairy tale. My parents' wedding album was my favorite—the pretty pictures perfectly sequenced to tell the story of my mother's perfect day. My mother with her parents. My mother and my granddad, looking handsome and slightly uncomfortable, before he walked her down the aisle. A wide-angle shot of the minister, the attendants and groomsmen, and the happy couple. Then there is a wonderful portrait of just my mother—she is glowing and looks beautiful in a demure, perfectly tailored off-white satin dress. She wore a pillbox hat (so Jackie Kennedy) with a delicate, tiny veil that shaded her olive skin like a bare shadow. On the next and final page is a picture of my parents in "leaving" clothes—my mother in a snappy travel suit with a fur-lined collar and a matching fur hat. It was a September wedding.

It's funny, but my mother and I rarely spoke of her afternoon wedding at a small country church on the outskirts of Winston-Salem, her experience as a bride or what I can only imagine would be the trials and tribulations of planning a wedding with

HER mother. But her wedding was imprinted on me nonetheless by way of that white, leather-bound wedding album. I'm not sure why, but I knew no funny stories of last-minute details, wedding-dress drama and pending calamity. She didn't offer up any lessons learned from her day in the sun. Strangely, I didn't ask. I thought I knew all I needed to know. And to this day, I could sit down with that book in hand and tell you MY VERSION of my mother's wedding day without turning a page.

This is the clueless naïveté that I brought to my own June wedding at a large city church in a breezy mountain North Carolina town. I had been a bridesmaid in more than a dozen weddings and endured extraordinary incidents of wedding-day woes, dress drama and obnoxious in-laws. While my wedding preferences were certainly informed by wedding etiquette tomes and five-pound bridal magazines, at the end of the day, that thirty-three-year-old, white, leather-bound photo album served as the unconscious linchpin of my wedding-day dreams.

I shared my deep-seated angst about not measuring up on my wedding day with my maid of honor, whose sole reason for being on the earth is to dedicate one full year of her life to my silly wedding drama and one full day of her life to trotting around behind me like a prissy, train-toting servant.

"Don't be silly," Suzanne said as we chatted by phone one winter day. "You're going to look great." She continued: "But come on, Char, you've been to as many weddings as I have, and you know, the bride ALWAYS looks gorgeous on her wedding day. It's karma, it's destiny, it's the order of all things good. The sun will always rise in the east and the bride will always look gorgeous on her wedding day. It's one of life's absolutes."

It took me a while to accept her theory, but she was right, of course. I wore a beautiful dress that only in retrospect did I note was eerily similar to my mother's. And like her, my hair was short and styled. My debut as a bride was wonderful—I felt pretty, happy and confident. Likewise, my mother dressed the part of stately, elegant mother of the bride and glided serenely down the aisle on the arm of my younger brother in an incredibly demure and age-appropriate dress that featured a beaded top and a pretty, flowing skirt in the most luscious shade of aquamarine. And Brad looked incredibly handsome in a simple black tux and white tie. He had more than dressed the part, and clearly come a long way since the early days of our engagement.

The spring that Brad proposed, he was getting dressed for one of our engagement parties—mutual work friends were hosting a cookout on the lake, complete with volleyball, beer and all things casual. I presented in a cute dress of some sort, with no intention of involving myself in any actual aspects of the cookout—it's not like I was going to really play volleyball; I assumed volleyball was for ambience only. You know, part of the "theme."

Standing in the hallway, freshly showered and ready to pick me up, was the love of my life, my future husband and father of my children, who was decked out in a dishwater-gray T-shirt, athletic shorts and high-top basketball shoes (with footie socks).

"You do know that you are the guest of honor at this event, right?" I asked, trying to suppress my horror at Brad's dress sense. After all, he was (and is) a swell guy.

"Sure," he responded. "Guest of honor at a cookout at the lake—hot dogs, beer, volleyball, the works."

"And you're going to wear that?" I asked. It came out before I knew what happened. In the blink of an eye, I had become every bad cliché about overbearing, opinionated and dictatorial girlfriends, despite the accent.

"Why not? It's a cookout and we're playing VOLLEYBALL."

It took all my restraint not to comment on why everything on his body was a bad idea, especially if one is dressing the part of guest of honor at an event that includes work colleagues, but I said no more and neither did he, and on we rolled. We arrived shortly before the majority of the guests (as guests of honor should do), hugged the hosts and grabbed a drink. The day was beautiful and the ambience was relaxed and fun. It was the perfect backdrop for a game of volleyball (or so I assumed since sundresses and volleyball don't mix), and my sporty fiancé immediately jumped on board. Our friends celebrated and toasted and we took lots of photos that would live on into posterity—with Brad in his grungy T-shirt and me in my cute ensemble.

The next day, though, as I tried to bask in the glow of our lovely little engagement gig, it was still niggling at me. Despite the very clear party "theme," I couldn't get over Brad's fashion choice, mostly because I knew he had some semblance of taste. Brad and I met at work and I had witnessed him cutting it beautifully in a dark worsted-wool suit. So why the disconnect?

"Listen," I said. "I just have to share something about yesterday and about how we're going to handle that kind of stuff for the next, oh, you know, fifty years."

We were in the den in my little bungalow in the heart of Charlotte. He sat on the couch patiently, ready for me to start. I fiddled with the very pretty ring that still felt new and clunky on my left hand and paced to and fro in front of the sofa, formulating my thoughts. I think he knew what was on my mind; sometimes it's like he's inside my head.

"You're thirty years old," I continued. "Way past the statute of limitations for wearing worn-out frat-party T-shirts and ratty gym shorts ANYWHERE, much less to a prewedding event, I don't care how casual it is. I was a little shocked and a bit bummed out." I paused, looking for any reaction that might tell me what I should say next. I got nothing. So I kept going.

"But you know what? I'm not going to be *that* girl. The one that is constantly riding your rear about what you're wearing. That's not how this is going to play out. I'm your fiancée, not your mother."

He just looked at me with a strangely neutral expression that lulled me into thinking he was listening to what I was saying. It was a trick he has come to master. I continued, not quite done.

"You're too smart not to know that when you dress like an overgrown frat boy who's too lazy to spiff up for people you respect and like, you get treated like an overgrown frat boy who's too lazy to spiff up for people he respects and likes. So by all means, keep on keeping on. But if you change your mind and want some input about how a thirty-year-old man dresses outside of work, I'd be happy to help. You're a handsome guy and you look great in some of your clothes and I'd like to see you wearing more of them. But I'm not going to browbeat you like you're a five-year-old every time we go out and you're dressed like Adam Sandler in some movie about emotionally stunted men. So, handsome, you just let me know, okay?"

Admittedly, it was a lofty and verbose speech that could have used a good edit. But Brad didn't freak out or stomp off in a huff. Rather he quietly processed some feedback that I had felt to be undeniably true—Brad knew how to dress the part and it meant a lot to me that he cared enough to do it. And after that, he did. Sure, some days were better than others. And still, on occasion, he asks for some input on which Brooks Brothers dress shirt goes best with his dozen pair of flat-front gabardine pants.

Like most people, Brad has his uniform, I have mine. It's important because it's about more than figuring out what looks good on you (though that's essential). It's also about figuring out what role you intend to play.

My sister-in-law Elise mentored a young woman who aspired to be an investment banker. Renee was incredibly competent (which meant she looked great on paper) but socially awkward (which meant she was a horrible interview). To add fuel to the fire, she dressed more like a dog groomer than an investment-banker-in-training. During Renee's first year at the bank, she alternated between two pairs of the exact same shoes—very sensible, wedgelike loafers, one pair in brown and the other black. Her third pair were tragic, turquoise-colored jelly flats that she wore on casual Fridays. Plastic shoes on Friday, in Renee's world, were part of her fashion code.

"Just when I thought it couldn't get any worse, it did," Elise commented on the day the plastic jelly shoes clickity-clacked across the trading floor. Elise, my smartly dressed, talented sister-in-law, had more on her hands than mentoring Renee in the art of Excel spreadsheets.

Are we judging Renee on her ability to dress the part? Yes, we are. Even Elise, an advocate for Renee, knew that her appearance was limiting her. Despite her solid work performance, her outward show and bearing were handicaps. Renee's success, as well as her mentor's, depended in some part on her ability to *look* the part. Was it outlined in the mentoring guidelines? No. Was it detailed in the job description? Of course not. So while it perhaps was un-PC and incredibly sexist (and likely not much talked about in the HR department), mentoring often bleeds into those gray areas. How do you approach a topic that can be so sensitive, so personal, so subjective?

"It wasn't really that subjective," Elise responded. "It was pretty obvious to most anyone that she needed to work on her presentation—her clothes, her hair, everything."

So Elise told Renee that she needed to try harder to dress the part, and encouraged her to be more professional in her appearance. "Look at the other women in the group," Elise suggested. "You don't have to dress like them. You don't have to be them. But take into account what they consider acceptable, and see what you can do." Renee was not offended, but seemed re-

Charla Muller

lieved to have someone acknowledge the blindingly obvious. So did she undergo a complete and utter transformation? Did she morph from the weird, bohemian egghead to the oh-so-lovely investment-banker swan? Is there a movie-of-a-week story waiting in the wings—the one where Renee dresses in head-to-toe Prada, closes the deal and wins the guy?

"Nope, didn't happen at all," said Elise. "But she was trying to dress the part. And it showed."

Shouldn't we get some brownie points for at least *trying* to dress the part? Trying to dress the part for Renee meant throwing out the plastic jelly shoes. Trying for a girlfriend in college was making sure her sweatpants weren't inside out before she headed to class.

So if we're all in the same league of *trying* to look good and working hard to dress the part, why aren't we more solicitous, more generous with our support, more open to offering compliments, to giving some props to our sisters—our harshest critics? Instead, when it comes to beauty and appearance, I think we're most often wounded by friendly fire.

A few years ago, I was prepping for a cooking segment on a local talk show in Charlotte. I had managed to parlay my fifteen minutes of fame as "the girl who wrote THAT book" into the girl who can pull off live cooking segments whenever the local producers are in a pinch. I was there to demo my aunt Yvonne's butterscotch pound cake, which is, and I am not exaggerating, obscenely over-the-top, "I could die happy right now" fabulous. I was dressing the part of author/cook in my funky patchwork apron. I found myself in the green room with Fannie Flagg,

214

author of *Fried Green Tomatoes* (as well as fourteen other fiction books, including the current one she was promoting) and a fixture on the game-show circuit in the seventies, including *The Match Game*. You should know that I LOVE Fannie Flagg. She is smart (a classically trained actress who has appeared both on stage and television), she is sassy (effortlessly holding her own against the Ricky Gervais of her era, Richard Dawson) and she is forever and graciously clever (stand-up comedienne, author and former Birmingham beauty queen and weather girl). She is all that and a bag of chips.

That day she looked FAB in a coral-colored suit with pretty pearl earrings and matching lip stain. She was charming to everyone in the green room, even those silly clods who had no earthly idea who she was. She tried my pound cake and I swooned with pride. She answered the rote and inane questions with composure and attentiveness. She said she was incredibly grateful to be invited on our little local talk show and couldn't wait, and I quote, "to come back." She was astute and chatty during commercial breaks and made the connection between my book and me. After the show, Fannie asked me about my experience and I shared with her that I'd never had such lovely fan mail and such appalling hate mail.

"Dawlin'," she said as she leaned into me and put her hand on mine. "Believe me, it doesn't matter what you do or how hard you try. Someone will always hate you." She looked at me with a soft and sincere gaze. "There is nothing you can do but keep on doing what you know how to do." I know . . . I was practically verklempt, too. I mean, I would have paid gobs of money to a therapist to hear those words over the years. Of course, there are plenty of reasons not to like me—I can be loud, opinionated and slightly oblivious to social cues when I've had too much wine, for example. While I've realized that I can't make everyone like me, I have spent the better part of four decades minding my manners, trying to put others first and essentially working hard to make sure people can't find a reason to hate me. But Fannie was absolutely right—it's a futile endeavor. Someone will always hate you. You can't control what others feel or think, but you can control how *you* feel and think. So dress the part you want to play, live it large and wear it well.

For a few years, I was dressing the part of Volunteer Mom and it was Wearing. Me. Out.

There is a Volunteer Mafia in every city. It's an underground syndicate that recruits and drafts unknowing women into its ranks and never lets them go. I had been a room mom at least a half dozen times (in fact, it has been rumored that my room-mom model had been franchised), chaired the board of the weekday school, served on the board of the PTA executive committee at the elementary school, baked pies, worked carpool line, managed a national preschool accreditation process and stuffed thousands of folders for back-to-school. In the spirit of full disclosure, this is considered a fairly manageable volunteer load in my Pretty City. I am not all that and a bag of chips when it comes to volunteering.

Likewise, I had learned what NOT to volunteer for, not based on the volunteer assignment du jour but on what I don't do well. And I don't do admin. It's true—not only do I stink at mundane administrative tasks, I loathe them.

"Char, sign up with me for the envelope-stuffing committee for the Children's Theater," one of my best pals, Kate, pleaded. "It only meets once a month for six months and we sit around and stuff and stamp five thousand envelopes. It will be fun to catch up."

Actually, it wouldn't be fun at all. And we wouldn't be able to catch up because my undiagnosed ADD would kick in and I'd get all agitated and wonder how stuffing, sealing and stamping five thousand envelopes could TAKE SO LONG. I'd rather die and come back as a receptionist at an infectious-disease medical practice. But thanks so much for thinking of me. I perform best with self-scheduled placements that don't require admin, manual labor or lots of meetings with silly women who natter on and on about which teacher they swore their child would never get, and how they relied on their private child-psychologist-cum-placement-counselor to write a letter to the principal about how Mary Sadie Elizabeth simply would not flourish in a first-grade classroom that didn't have full light for eight hours and a teacher who didn't speak Mandarin Chinese. Nope, I don't mix well with those volunteers. And I can bond with my pal Kate over wine anytime, as she does none of that nattering and is actually loads of fun.

But for every opportunity that I politely declined with a "thank you, but I'm not feeling called to help coordinate the delivery of 482 home-baked pies to the school the day before

Thanksgiving break so we can package them with a ribbon and special handwritten card, and distribute them to the entire teaching staff as a sign of our Thanksgiving gratitude," the more I got asked. Didn't these people know that I was AT CAPACITY? Didn't they know that when I said no to them, it was because someone else caught me at a weak moment and I said yes to them? Didn't they see what a hot mess I was? Did they not KNOW that my house was a wreck, my laundry was stacked to the ceiling, I was stepping over cat barf and that my mother was keeping a tally of my unreturned phone calls?

That's when I realized that my attempts to dress the part about 30 percent of the time of a fairly well-pulled-together working mom who had things somewhat under control was leading people to think, of all things, that I *was* a fairly well-pulled together working mom who had things somewhat under control. When nothing could have been further from the truth.

Perhaps I needed to dress the part of Working Mom on the Verge of a Nervous Breakdown Who Always Has a Standing Rezzie at the "Spa" with the White Padded Rooms. Perhaps if I looked completely ragged out, acted crazy and irritable and never washed my hair, people would keep their distance. I know I would steer clear of me. I thought about staging some "incidents" around town to help lend momentum to my campaign to exit the Volunteer Mafia. It crossed my mind that I could show up hung over to teach Sunday school. Drive erratically in the carpool line while checking e-mail. Send in inedible and rancid goodies to the bake sale. But then I realized that not only did that feel a little extreme, it would take energy and planning to dress the part of crazy, too.

I said no, I swear I did, just not enough. And sometimes it would be too late. Such as when the Volunteer Mafia wants to take you to lunch to "discuss" an incredible opportunity to work together—that's when you're hosed. Because once you're seated at your favorite little bistro nibbling on mesclun with grilled salmon, it's too late. You can't say no; they are treating you to lunch, after all. Your other choices are to enter the Witness Protection Program and go into hiding until people think you are dead, or check into said spa with the white padded room. Even my mother was in a state of disbelief.

"You are on the go from sunup until sundown and NEVER available by phone," she commented one day by said phone as I was lamenting my chaotic schedule and she was conjuring up some fabulous piece of art in her sunny patio home in her lush, green, gated Florida community.

"You have too much on your plate. I don't care how 'fun' this stuff seems at the time or how flattered you are to be asked, you have GOT to start saying no more often." This from the woman whose daily productivity exceeded that of a Third World country. And she has great jewelry. But she was right. Again.

It had gotten to a point where I needed to train myself to get out of these situations that were stretching me thin. So I would practice in front of the mirror in my bedroom, pushing and pulling my lips to form the two-letter word over and over and over. "Nooooo. Nooooo. Nooooo."

"What are you doing?" Brad asked one evening when he saw me massaging my mouth.

"I'm practicing saying nooooo," I garbled as my hands mushed my face. I turned to him. "Noooo. What do you think?"

"You're kidding, right? You have no problem saying no."

"I'm trying to get better at saying no to the right things, okay?" I quipped.

"Okay, sure," he said. "Have you called the repair guy about our leaky roof?"

I turned to him. "Noooooooooo."

So instead of dressing the part of a crazed working mom who couldn't be trusted with a volunteer assignment, entering the Witness Protection Program or blurting out "Noooooo" before anyone could approach me at church, school or the Rite-Aid, I had another idea.

The Volunteer Résumé Bracelet.

The VRB stores all of your volunteer experience—past and current—in a little chip embedded in a trendy cuff, à la Wonder Woman. And other VRBs can access it. So when a mom approached me in the parking lot of the grocery store regarding those eighteen voice-mail messages she left me asking for an update on my prayerful consideration of leading the arrangements committee next fall for the women's welfare league (not their real name), I can flash my cool cuff and stop that overbearing volunteer in her tracks.

"Charla!" she would exclaim. "I'm so embarrassed! I had no IDEA how booked you are! You're involved in so much—you're an incredible mother, neighbor, sister, wife, community member, marketing professional, advocate for the underserved and all-around thoughtful friend. How in the world do you do it all? I bow at the feet of the Volunteer Queen whose hair looks très shiny and well conditioned, by the way. A thousand pardons for disturbing you." And she would leave me alone and I would keep dressing the part . . . of me. Which, depending on the day, could be marketing consultant heading to lunch in a snappy sweater set; carpool mom heading into the Siberian tundra for her three-hour carpool gig and armed with sustenance, comfortable shoes and lots of lip balm; or happy volunteer to select causes that draw out her passion and enthusiasm.

Dressing the part is an amalgamation of a lot of things—appreciation for what wears well, awareness of what the part entails and an ability to adapt and to flex. And equally important, we have to decide if dressing for certain parts is even in our DNA. Because it doesn't matter if you're an up-and-coming banker, an author/baker or a volunteer refugee on the lam. At the end of the day, we should all unapologetically live out the part. And dressing the part will follow.

(And patent pending on the Volunteer Résumé Bracelet.)

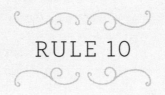

RULE 10

Looks Fade,
Be Interesting

When my sister-in-law Elise turned forty, I helped plan a birthday beach weekend with some of her besties. It was low-key and filled with all of her favorites—great wine and appetizers, downtime with friends, walks along the shore, a decadent custom-made birthday cake that could send one into a diabetic coma and even a private, early-morning yoga session on the beach. Elise had friends from high school, college and work as well as me, at forty-four, the elder stateswomen of the weekend. September at the beach is a beautiful time of year and the seven of us settled into my parents' beach house to enjoy it.

We kicked off our first full day on the beach with a yoga session. I'm not a yoga groupie, but I was fully embracing anything my awesome sister-in-law so desired. The beach was deserted that morning and Janine, our instructor, had the seven of us spread across a large swath of packed sand, fully engaged in Standing Eagle. The sun was peeking over the sand dunes and it was a serene, peaceful session. Until we hit Downward Dog and I made the mistake of opening my eyes and looking back up at my legs. From this horrifying vantage point I witnessed my knees doing something I had never seen them do before.

Falling.

There was only one thing I could think: *Et tu, Brute?*

Of all body parts that I knew would betray me, I wasn't prepared for my KNEES. I was managing through the wrinkles and sunspots from my lack of sunscreen discipline. I was okay with the fact that my feet had never regained their prepregnancy shape and size and were now a full size bigger. And my dimpled thighs were alive and well and jiggling right along. But I never thought I would have to contend with knees that sagged, stretched and looked like a sixth-grade papier-mâché topographical map—ill-formed and lumpy.

I shut my eyes, focused on my breathing and then imagined myself wearing nothing but full-length pants for the rest of my days. But I couldn't actually do that. Really, full-length pants are impractical, especially down south during the dog days of summer. So, as I moved into another pose, I resigned myself to the cold, hard truth that in addition to my sagging chest and tush, which can be camouflaged, lifted and contained with a bra and Spanx, there was no such thing as an underwire knee bra or a knee girdle. Yet.

My friends and our knees are hitting our mid-to-late forties now. And while we might "feel" like this is the best time of our lives—we are cranking in a career, our kids are no longer sleep-stealing toddlers, we're getting volunteer commitments under control—we can't dispute the fact that we are closer to fifty than to twenty-five.

Nonetheless, when Brad and I received an invite to a joint fiftieth birthday party for Ava and Mary Anne, hosted by their husbands, I was shocked. If I had friends celebrating five decades on this planet, that meant I was somewhere in the ballpark, too, right? But what really struck me was that Ava and Mary Anne didn't look anywhere close to fifty. Perhaps it had something to do with the fact that they had kids a bit later in life, but they are fit, sporty and youthful. Or perhaps they've just been living right—schedules and workloads that allow them the opportunity to play tennis, make their favorite hot-yoga class, manage a facial schedule and access some great hair colorists. Of course, I was happy to be invited to what I knew would be a really fun soiree, sure.

It wasn't going to be a surprise party. Even though Ava's and Mary Anne's husbands were listed as the hosts, they planned the whole thing. Which made for a great time. Overall, I don't think most women liked to be surprised—at least in that way. Some diamond earrings? An evening out to a favorite restaurant? An offer to take the cat to the vet? Sure. Of course. How lovely. Please do.

But surprises that involve birthdays, lots of people, a cute outfit and some serious grooming considerations—and catering? Nope. We need to know and we need to be prepared. Brad never really believes me when I tell him this.

"I'm not kidding, hon," I told him when we were discussing

Ava and Mary Anne's party on our way to the mountains to visit my parents. The kids were settled in the backseat; giant earphones eclipsed their ears as they watched a movie. As we wound our way up Saluda Mountain, I made my case.

"When I declare that under no circumstances would I ever, *ever* want a surprise party of any kind, I am not hinting, bluffing or playing hard to get. Really. I don't want one. Nothing would make me more miserable." I turned to him for confirmation that he heard me loud and clear. Brad just sat there silently, eyes on the road, right eyebrow cocked. It was obvious he didn't quite believe me.

"I'm not telling you one thing and then sending you some secret mind-meld willing you to do the exact opposite, hon," I insisted. "Please trust me when I tell you this. No. Surprise Parties. Ever." He so didn't believe me then, which keeps me in a constant state of surprise-party panic now. So I settled back into my bucket seat and texted a girlfriend to confirm what she was going to wear to the party that was only a few weeks away.

It was a casual, outdoor celebration with a bartender, lots of nice catered food and plenty of alcohol for girls like me, who simply couldn't wrap our heads around this number *fifty*. I needed to wander aimlessly around the lovely party, constantly refreshing my drink and laboring on and on *and on* about the fact that all these beautiful people couldn't be teetering on the brink of the second half of life. I know, I found myself boorish, too.

Mary Anne's husband was the drummer in the band that played, and they were perched on a small, makeshift stage in the back corner of the yard. The band performed songs that showed everyone's age: Van Morrison, the Eagles, Squeeze.

"They're having too much fun to not know they're not that good," Brad whispered in my ear as he approached me from behind and slid his arm around my waist.

"And everyone else is having too much fun to care," I said as I raised my glass in tribute, swaying back and forth. We both watched people dance to old music that tricked us into feeling young. Music is sneaky that way.

Ava and Mary Anne looked terrific. Mary Anne kissed several of the male guests square on the lips as they departed. It was her birthday, there was champagne and she was turning fifty, after all. I was both appalled and impressed with her half-century brazenness. And it made me wonder, was Mary Anne now a cougar? She seemed too young, too sassy, too much of a pretty peer.

But then again, Anne Bancroft, the Mother of All Cougars, was thirty-six when cast in the role of Mrs. Robinson for the film *The Graduate*. That a thirty-something woman would qualify as an older woman is laughable today. In fact, imagine the talent pool from which to recruit a modern-day Mrs. Robinson. We don't have enough beautifully manicured fingers and toes on which to count the number of hip, great-looking, middle-aged women who look half their age. They are as ubiquitous a fixture in today's world as smartphones and belly rings.

Which means life as a cougar is not the exception but the expectation. Isn't it just so great that "older" women have the means, the technology and the ability to make themselves look and feel years younger? Youth is wasted on the young, so some of us get a do-over. A do-over that we can orchestrate at forty, fifty or sixty. It feels like an interruption of the time-space continuum that could impact the proper order of things, but who am I to complain about the incredible access to potions, procedures and paints that can make me look at forty-five better than I ever did at thirty-five? The problem is that I'm not sure what to do or what I'm willing to do that I'm not already doing. Do I tackle my negatives (like my knees) or continue to accentuate my positives (like my hair)?

These last few years, I visit Rob monthly. It wasn't my bob, which was motoring along at whatever speed Rob chose, but my roots. Everyone in my family was more salt than pepper before they turned forty. My younger brother looks hip and interesting. My dad, who is completely snow white, looks notably distinguished. My mother and I? Well, I can't tell you how we look because as sure as a Lancôme free gift with purchase, we will never live to see that day. So every four weeks or so I'm visiting the Bob Whisperer.

One day I noticed the stylist working the chair next to Rob. The stylist who has a really dramatic white streak in the front. It was striking and a tad mysterious. A white streak wouldn't interfere with the Bob Whisperer's bob juju, I thought; it would simply enhance it, while also paying homage to my roots' roots. Perhaps draw attention away from the knees, you know?

I tucked that little idea away with a note to self to ask Rob about it at my next appointment. In the meantime, fate shined on my well-conditioned head in the form of a serendipitous trip to Ulta. There, tucked in the corner of the discount bin at checkout was a white, clip-in hair extension—the perfect aid to test my glamorous white streak theory. It was about six inches long and had a little comb at the end. I bought it and that evening, I "inserted" my white streak, positioned it as a long, cool swipe of bangs, and went about my business. My mother, who was visiting at the time from Florida, walked into the house with both of my kids in tow.

I was sitting on the couch, working on a stylish nonchalance for my "mysteriously sophisticated white streak" debut. They noticed immediately.

"Ewwww, what's that in your hair?" my son blurted out as he came closer to inspect it.

"Mo-hom, what have you done now?" chided my daughter.

My mother just grinned. This was the woman who wore some seriously freaky-fab-frosted wigs in the seventies, after all, and liked to come home from the hairdresser and "trim" up her cut with a mirror and twenty-year-old manicure scissors. The woman was fearless when it came to hair, so I knew she would at least appreciate the effort.

But even the Christopher Columbus of Coiffures gave it the boot. "No, hon, that will not work. For starters, it changes your entire skin tone. You'll have to buy all new makeup."

Brad was more succinct. "I don't like it. You look like Cruella de Vil."

I didn't even take the idea back to the Bob Whisperer. We all know his response, now, don't we? That's why we pay people like Rob the Bob Whisperer the big bucks. In the midst of this weird battle against aging, I pay Rob to save me from myself.

Like most who are hustling to stave off the inevitable march of time, I'm challenged with the elusive Getting Pretty Tipping Point. Three years ago, I was traveling with two women whose husbands work with Brad. We were on a plane to California, happy to be invited along on a business trip. We were kibitzing about cute shoes, clothes that travel well and exercise classes. All this chatter led to Lani's story about a friend of a friend who was a self-absorbed narcissist.

Well, she didn't call her a self-absorbed narcissist (which is totally redundant), but I'm trying to make a point. Anyway, this friend of a friend runs exactly sixty-five minutes every morning, every day of the year, at the exact time, at the exact same pace, come rain, sleet or snow. She then must bathe, coif and dress impeccably for her day. She obsesses about her diet, her clothes, her hair and her ability to wear short-shorts (how can her knees NOT be sagging?). She wears formfitting clothes that make mundane chores difficult. Apparently it's hard to vacuum the den in six-inch Stuart Weitzman wedges.

"She's so obsessed with looking young and current that it never occurs to her that she looks silly and sad," Lani solemnly noted. "Plus, her sisters get pissed every year at the beach because she's always exercising, showering, primping and adhering to some hyper-regimented schedule, while they're cooking, cleaning and managing a beach-house-full of kids and husbands, including hers."

At what point does the quest for and commitment to pretty tip into one-dimensional, hyperfocused self-absorption? I imagine most rational gals (and I consider myself one on most days) struggle with the balance of too much and not enough when it comes to getting pretty. We know there are things that trump flawless skin, firm décolletage and perfectly positioned highlights. We know on a deeper level that much of pretty extends beyond the façade and that vacuous, self-centered people who spend their days polishing their veneer and have no appreciation for their interior or the interiors of others could very truly be the end of humanity as we know it.

As my friends and I nurse tennis injuries, ego injuries, sagging knees and crow's-feet, we find ourselves fully entrenched in this aging battle and no longer linger on the outskirts of the battlefield. Is it possible to win the battle without losing ourselves?

While in California, Lani and I connected with Trish. I didn't know Trish very well, even though I had socialized with her a few times a year for the past six or seven years at various business functions with my husband. While I was clearly the wife of a junior woodchuck and she clearly sat at the top of the pecking order at these events, she was always warm and engaging and remembered to ask about my children. Trish lived on the West Coast and had been married for many years to a very dashing, very trim and very successful man. They have many daughters and lots of grandchildren. I imagined Trish lived a very social, well-traveled and glamorous life. I just know that she hobnobbed and cocktailed with some seriously fun and interesting folks. Despite the fact that her daughters are nearly my age, it didn't occur to me that she might be the age of my parents. She was California pretty in a beachy, natural way—she wore funky glasses, sported interesting jewelry and showed none of the typical "signs" of work. Scars embedded in her hairline. Fish lips. Eyes stretched to the breaking point. Anytime I could connect with Trish, I tried. It was if she was a talisman on aging well and I wanted a bit of it to rub off on me.

"Women today, they're just silly! This is what you need to look good," she said one evening over cocktails at a beautiful home on 17-Mile Drive that overlooked the Pacific Ocean. I leaned in, along with the other women standing in our small circle, and listened hard. She raised her left hand and numbered off her pearls of wisdom. "A good pair of boots, well-tailored clothes that don't show your arms, some Latisse, and a book club. Oh, and go to church, for God's sake."

I let that sink in, running each one through my own personal pretty screen. The other women did, too. I could see us all processing, calculating and assessing. It was a surprisingly honest moment. I asked a passing waiter for another drink. One woman went to get a wrap for her arms. Trish's daughter smiled in knowing agreement. There you have it, gals, from the lips of a Beauty Jedi who's lived enough years to speak such truths.

Later, I asked about the Book Club—and church.

"Women need a book club or something like it—it makes you interesting," Trish said while she helped herself to a beautiful piece of sashimi tuna from a tray passed by a handsome waiter. "And church? Who doesn't need something that makes you realize the world is so not about you, so why not get off your duff and go help someone?"

Why indeed? Read, help others, connect with God, be interesting. That doesn't seem so hard, does it?

Because we all have adorably gorgeous friends who dazzle simply by showing up. And well-packaged cohorts who spend HOURS talking about their beauty regimen. Or colleagues who spent half their paycheck at Sephora and the other half at Spray Me Tan USA. Is it too late for them? Is it too late to learn Mandarin Chinese? Start a foundation to save some species of endangered monkeys? Start collecting Art Deco chandeliers? Of course not.

My mother has all sorts of collections—Sallie Middleton watercolor botanicals, Royal Stafford porcelain flower bouquets, sterling-silver candlesticks, Herend figurines (preferably, but not always, rabbits), antique demitasse cup-and-saucer sets, Timmy Woods handbags. The list goes on and on, really.

"Always collect something," my mother counsels. "It gives you something to do and something to pass on. And," she adds with emphasis, "people always have an idea of something to buy for you." I contend that my mother is passing down along with her collections a deeply rooted southern truth: collect something, anything—art, beer-bottle openers, husbands, friends—as it makes you more interesting. And if it doesn't, at least it gives you something to do. And if you're not getting a good lineage passed down to you, forty-eight place settings of Towle sterling-silver flatware should bring a bit of comfort. So if beauty fades, lead-crystal brandy snifters and the art of conversation about said lead-crystal brandy snifters are forever, aren't they?

Collections do indeed make us more interesting, and collecting people is no exception. Southerners are terribly astute at this—it's part of our genetic makeup. What started out as a survival skill—are you a Hatfield or a McCoy (aka a friend or a foe)?—later morphed into a highly attuned ability to place people, to rank position and to identify pedigree. "Where are you from?" is just another form of a calling card down here—it's an opportunity to get to know you and to determine how much more we would like to get to know you. When used properly, it's an engaging way to make connections, to find common interests and associations, to make acquaintances. To be interesting. Most important, if done well, it can make you a charming and highly sought-after dinner party guest. As in, "You mean your first cousin's husband who is from Birmingham roomed with my brother at Woodberry? Well, that's wund-dah-ful! Let's be friends for-ev-ah! Are you free for drinks next week?" When used for evil, it can be patronizing, condescending and boorish. And quickly slot you as a D-level dinner-party guest. As in, "Oh dear, you mean to tell me that you're from the Middle Tennessee Keanes? The ones that are kin to that senator who was found bound and naked in that interstate bathroom? My, where is Mary Martha? If you'll excuse me, I need to cancel cocktails for next week."

Even better than stuff, my grandfather, being an interesting gentleman, collected people—his obituary proudly claimed that he knew more than five thousand, all of them by their first name. No one mentioned how many actually attended the funeral, but legend has it that they spilled out of the church into the street. A collection that lived on posthumously, as all good collections do, in an incredible attribute he passed along to my father. The art of being interested.

To state the obvious, part of being interesting is simply showing an interest in others. I had an old boss who taught me the power of this simple precept.

Never married, Edwina had family money, connections and smarts. She hired me at a PR agency in Atlanta when I was in my twenties, and couldn't have been more interested in me not just as a new hire but, oddly enough, as a person. She was handsome in a well-bred sort of way, not so much pretty but rather coolly elegant. She wore tasteful jewelry, expensive and well-tailored suits and luscious silk scarves. She asked smart questions and sparked engaging conversation around everything from my family (she discovered she was a contemporary of my father's) to my hometown (her family had a vacation home there) to my old job (she wanted to know all about how things were done at New York agencies) to how I was settling down in Atlanta (she gave me a thumbs-up on my Buckhead rental house and offered some restaurant suggestions). Anyone outside the South might find this intrusive and off-putting, but having just returned to the South from Manhattan, I found it warm and encouraging, kind of like cozying up under a familiar quilt after spending a long day in brisk, cold weather. I found Edwina easy to talk to, conversant in lots of fun topics outside of work. In other words, I found her lovely and interesting.

Many years later, I spotted her at a social function in another state. She was seated at a table across the room, deeply engrossed in conversation. While I only worked one year for Edwina, she made a lasting impression on me, so I didn't hesitate to make my way over to her, fully prepared to reintroduce myself. After all, how many twenty-something single professional gals had marched through the hallways of her firm over the years? The minute I said my name, a warm smile enveloped her face. She took my hand in hers and started peppering me with questions. She was delighted to see me, she wanted to know about all I had been doing and she wanted to introduce me to her family.

"I would love to call you the next time I'm in Atlanta," I offered up as we were winding down.

"Indeed, it would be an onah to have you in my home," she offered in a rich female southern baritone. That's exactly how she said it, I swear.

"Indeed, it would be an onah to have you in my home."

And I would love nothing more than to visit Edwina in her home, because I discovered she actually lived in the Four Seasons Hotel in midtown Atlanta. I mean, who does that—besides über-wealthy Manhattan investment bankers? Edwina, that's who. While she had all the external trappings of a really lovely life, she had all the internal trappings as well.

One of the gifts of maturity (which often does not correlate with age) is an appreciation for the delicate balance between internal and external pretty. It's a universal truth—external beauty fades, knees sag and tummies stretch, despite the incredible weapons we now have to beat back the beast of aging. But internal pretties have a much longer shelf life and allow us a more gratifying opportunity to be not just pretty, but pretty interesting.

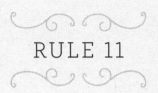

RULE 11

Age with Grace
and Die with Poise

Some call it "the Candy Shop" because there is always something new and delicious to try—a flat prepregnancy belly postbaby, taut dewy skin, pouty lips, wide-open eyes. Every time I walk through the halls of my dermatologist's office, my sweet (and savvy) anesthetist whispers in my ear all the way to her small room—pointing out the new goodies proudly on display. Look, Janine just had the new Pumpkin Peel. Karen has been using Latisse. Mandy did Botox and Restylane. Camille had a boob job and brow-lift.

"Don't they look wonderful?" she asks. I'm not sure . . . what did they look like before?

It's hard to even pick an octogenarian out of the crowd these days, what with hair extensions, lips inflated to the size of life preservers, new tops and bottoms, spider-like Rogaine eyelashes and big honkin' sunglasses. We're witness to the first generation of Freeze-Dried Aging—seeing for the first time how tattoos, body piercings, bolt-on breasts, hair extensions and oversize lips look on the over-seventy crowd, and preliminary reports suggest it ain't pretty. Can too much liposuction drain one's dignity as well as one's belly fat?

Lani thinks so. Lani lives on a horse farm out in the country. She has a thick strawberry-blond bob, funky glasses that can't hide her inquisitive eyes and an athlete's figure still at fifty-something. Her slightly tomboyish patina lends itself to riding boots and jeans as well as a sheath dress and chic Tory Burch flats. She talks about her friends, some of whom are getting face-lifts and all sorts of work done.

"It's alarming. For God's sake, you have to give me a heads-up. It's just not polite to debut your 'new work' without any warning at all," she said.

"I was at a dinner party recently and another guest arrived. It was so obvious that she had some extreme face work done. She didn't mention it, so we didn't mention it, but it so obviously needed mentioning and it was all just incredibly awkward."

Then the story got even better. Another dinner guest—a prominent plastic surgeon—came over and whispered to Lani and her cohorts, "Just to let you know, that is not my work."

"I mean, that's how BAD it was," Lani said. "A plastic surgeon needed to caveat the poor girl's work."

I agreed. Plastic surgery is the new elephant in the living room. Surely there are etiquette guidelines out there to help people through proper protocol when friends and family embark on elective surgery that can impact others' ability to recognize them. Should there be an announcement? A sign-up sheet for meals? Do we host a "sip and see" much like we do to show off new babies? Can we ask if this was elective surgery or rather a new approach to the Witness Protection Program?

So in addition to an occasional visit with Botox or a weird desire to experiment with hair extensions, I cast the occasional shout-out to my pretty peeps to see if they have discovered the Fountain of Youth in their (firm) neck of the woods. Since I'm secretly convinced they'll find it in California, I yearn to stalk Susan, my Malibu Barbie college roommate, who lives outside L.A. in Manhattan Beach. I just KNEW that she was keeper of the latest and greatest beauty breakthroughs.

> CHARLA TEXT: On treadmill watching infomercial on Dr. Perricone. He says it's not too late for beautiful skin AND that there is hope for my neck, too. What should I do? Is Dr. Perricone so last year in LA?

> CHARLA TEXT: Up late, can't sleep. Cindy Crawford looks incredible. Should I check out Meaningful Beauty? I swear it looks like she has had NO work done. Is that even possible? Is she a genetic freak? Do you think she's nice? She seems nice. I hope she's nice.

> CHARLA TEXT: At Costco, they sell StriVectin, that neck wattle cream. Do you think it works? Do you even have a wattle yet? Text me your wattle and I'll text you mine.

Of course, no one really has the answers. So I did nothing, kept on using my drugstore moisturizer and cleanser with occasional rotations of Obagi and Retin-A (when I remembered), and kept my eyes peeled for any pretty peers with great-looking knees.

Aging is tricky, but so is dying, and there are examples everywhere of people doing both with fabulous flair as well as fabulous desperation. Everyone wants to live forever . . . or at least long *enough* (and who's to say exactly how long that is?). While southerners are a scrappy breed and fighting death is a natural human tendency, even my grandmother was conflicted. She was mad about dying and irritated by living. "Burying all your friends gets old and making new ones is too much trouble," she once told me. My mother's people live forever regardless of their best efforts and my grandmother hung on until she was ninety-four. My own mother could likely slug bourbon and smoke a pack of unfiltered Camels daily (neither of which she does) and still live to be a hundred years old (and be quite cranky about it).

My father, on the other hand, wakes up every day amazed—stunned, really—that he is STILL ALIVE, having outlived every member of his family (save his wife, children and a few nephews and a niece) and outsmarting and outworking all sorts of genetic ills and grievances. He does yoga, gets regular massages, eats right, meets with his personal trainer, reads constantly and often carries his own clubs when he walks eighteen holes. What's given my dad this kind of energy and discipline? Well, besides the daily miracle of waking up, I think it's the Bubble.

The Bubble is the little slice of heaven my parents have called home for nearly half the year for the last decade. I call it the Bubble because everything is better inside this little cocoon of paradise. The sky really is bluer, the grass is greener, the flowers are brighter and people really are happier inside the gilded gates of this golf community. Landscapers buzz around in golf carts from sunup to sundown, sporting pith helmets and tending to every form of plant life on their beautiful campus. Residents ride their bikes to golf, yoga, tennis and bridge, and set off a brisk ring of their bike bell and a jaunty "on your left" alert as they pass you. While I could never fast-forward far enough to actually imagine my parents settling into a gated community where identical patio homes and condos line palm-tree-lined streets and cul-de-sacs named after birds, they have done just that. They love their pretty house on Meadowlark Lane as well as their new friends on Egret Drive and on Sanderling Circle. And after I visited, I realized my parents were rocking. My dad is playing some of the best golf of his life in a community that caters to outstanding senior golfers. My mother has taken up painting and now exhibits at shows and paints on commission. They have made new friends who have similar interests and they like to go to concerts and museums. They get lots of vitamin D.

But fab little gated warm-weather communities don't have the market cornered on gracious aging—they just have an unusually high concentration of folks who are doing it well. I contend they're everywhere, if you know where to look. The first time I meet Mrs. Neal I was struck by two things. The first was her size. She is tiny, like a dancer. I pictured her running ahead a few steps and launching into an effortless grand jeté. The second was her hair—a thick, vivid white, cut in a short pageboy and girlishly pulled back from her face with a drugstore barrette.

I was at Mrs. Neal's house to have some clothes altered. This was years before I was introduced to Marine Sergeant Marie. I didn't mind waiting in her sitting room, which is off the kitchen and festooned with Christmas decorations (even in the middle of March when I was there), handmade needlepoint pillows, small porcelain figurines and a stack of magazines, including a 1975 *Bon Appétit*. I sat patiently on a settee as tiny as she was, grateful for a quiet moment, facing her fireplace draped in faux holly.

Soon she is ready for me. "I am glad to meet you. Alison said you might come," she says, in a light European accent. When I stood, I realized she was the size of my daughter when she was eleven. She took my hands into hers and looked up at me. Her eyes were bright and unflinching. Her face, wide and welcoming. There was a long pause, which made me wonder if I had food in my teeth. She finally broke the silence.

"I have an ability to know the good from the bad," she said. Her eyes intently scanned my eyes and my face, looking for clues I could not fathom. Was she looking for good fashion taste? Good credit? Good teeth?

Apparently satisfied, she squeezed my hand and said, "I can tell you are good. Let's get started." And she turned and walked down the narrow hall to a back bedroom that was home to her antique Singer and tall racks that hold clothes that don't fit people. On the way, her snow-white hair bobbed up and down—she could have been a schoolgirl in silhouette. I followed her.

She continued, apparently unfazed by my surprised silence in response to her extraordinary introduction.

"I was ten when I went to the camps. I had to learn right away who was good and who was bad. It was a helpful skill to learn." She turned to face me and smiled broadly. "Now, what are we doing today?"

I was riveted. Mrs. Neal, who, at nearly eighty, scurried around on her hands and knees around my feet, pins in her pursed little mouth, hemming up pants that were too long (pants that would forever and ever be too long, I might add), chatting about the length, the weather, her neighbors. I was dazzled into silence by the lilt of her voice, by her small, graceful stature, by her beautiful face and most of all by her confident pronouncement of my goodness. She was encouraging, making recommendations on how to take in a jacket, to best make a hem, to sew up a pocket.

When I left, she patted my hand and said. "You are pretty, like Alison. A good girl." Her glow, despite her age (or perhaps because of it), shone bright and it seemed to have rubbed off on me. I carried it home to my family and that night at dinner shared with them my first encounter with Mrs. Neal. They, too, were captivated.

My children wanted to meet her, eager to capture some of her glow. A pretty glow that came from an inherent warmth and compassion. I can only assume that the reason Mrs. Neal can pinpoint goodness in others is because she has it in such abundance herself. An important lesson as we all search for the secrets to pretty.

As we age, some people, like my parents, head to Florida to

find their glow. Some, like Mrs. Neal, pass along their glow. And then there are others who want to suck the glow out of everyone with their uncensored opinions and general crankiness. My parents call it "losing your governor." The term refers to the absence of that little voice inside our heads that keeps our manners, opinions and commentary in check. Reaching a certain age earns you the privilege of relaxing or losing your governor, thereby granting you a freedom to say things that are blunt, occasionally offensive and often true.

No, I don't want any more of your damn breakfast casserole, Marge. Your cooking stinks, it's a miracle I'm not dead already.

I don't know what happened to Sue Anne's children. She married that smart doctor and moved to Raleigh. But her children are dumb as trees and neither one got her looks. So much for that.

Don't let Ronald fool you. He's tight as a tick and mean as a snake. And standing on the church steps every Sunday handing out programs for the eleven o'clock service doesn't change a thing.

Oh, honey, didn't you know? Your mother always loved your sister more than you. Why do you think she left her the sterling-silver tea service and you your father's commemorative shot-glass collection?

And of course, as we age, we often lose our fashion governor, too. I have mixed emotions about this. On the one hand, I appreciate the joie de vivre that comes with a newfound fashion freedom. I mean, that whole red hat gig isn't really my thing, but I appreciate and support the sentiment. But there is a big difference, as we've discussed, between throwing fashion caution to the wind and just not trying. Case in point, my mother-in-law.

I pulled in the driveway one afternoon in my big honkin' SUV and spotted Anne on the side porch, stretched across an outdoor chair and ottoman, noodling her way through, I assumed, her daily *New York Times* crossword puzzle. It was a teacher workday and she had graciously offered to hang out with the kids. My mother-in-law looked younger than seventy-two in her very trim size-six blue jeans and a cute top. Then I glanced down. And I noted, with slight surprise and a little horror, the thick, white athletic socks and brown, open-toed Clarks leather slide sandals. You read that right—thick, white athletic socks and brown, open-toed Clarks leather slide sandals. It was a total disconnect for this youthful woman who regularly kayaks and plays tennis every few weeks. And you know how I feel about feet. I just had to say something about her lack of a fashion governor. I unloaded the car and greeted her on the porch. After some small talk, I made a segue.

"Anne," I said, choosing my words carefully. "I'm sorry if this puts you on the spot, but I have GOT to address what the heck you have going on with your shoes." She looked up at me from her newspaper, squinting her hazel eyes, and waited for more.

"Please," I implored. "You cannot wear white sweat socks with brown leather, open-toed, slip-on sandals. If your feet are cold, wear socks and shoes. If your feet are hot, wear shoes or sandals, but no socks. You are too young and too hip to go shuffling around town with that kind of footgear." Pause. "Anne, you're better than that."

She glanced down at her feet with a small, sheepish grin. She knew I was right. But she wasn't ready to completely throw in the towel.

"You know, this is what everyone was wearing on my trip," she offered up in reference to her recent travels. Oh, she's good, that one.

"Yes, Anne, in CHINA, everyone wears thick white socks and slide-on sandals. BUT, we're not in China now, okay? So how about some fashion assimilation on this side of the planet?"

She threw her head back and laughed, a tacit acknowledgment of my point. And the next time I saw her she was sporting brown, open-toed Clarks leather slide sandals with thin, navy trouser socks. Touché.

Part of aging with grace is keeping a close eye on our internal and external pretty governors. And while it is quite all right to retire some of our external pretty habits, it's worth a quick gut check to confirm that our internal pretty habits are still firmly in place. And if you're like some of my pretty heroes who focus on book clubs, church, volunteering, collecting things, spotting goodness in others and taking up new hobbies, I suspect no one will even notice. Because pretty will be less about what we may no longer choose or be able to present on the outside and more about how freakin' fabulous we present from the inside. Which, for the women who paid attention and put in the practice, means pretty awesome.

My grandmother's funeral was held on a breezy September day in the same country church where she had served as a member of the choir for fifty years. While in the choir, rarely did she need a hymnal or a songbook—you would be hard-pressed to find a hymn my grandmother did not know by heart. In a nod to tradition, it was an open-casket funeral—a first for both my husband and children. Where I'm from, open-casket funerals are de rigueur, and since we're all voyeurs at heart, the "viewing" offers us one last chance to check out the newly deceased. Even in death, we want to make sure everyone looks pretty. While my husband and children found it unsettling, I found it comforting. She looked pretty in a way that felt familiar to me.

Her grandchildren spoke of her incredible faith, quirky sense of humor and superb cast-iron-skillet corn bread. We sang her favorite hymns, including "Great Speckled Bird." The service ended with a video clip of an interview the minister conducted with my grandmother a year or so prior as part of a church-wide anniversary celebration. It was a short clip and, like my grandmother, to the point. In it, she articulated what she thought of her life, how and why she lived it and what she hoped for her five generations of family. It was a jarring moment—to see on a screen the "live" version of the person who actually lay in the coffin in front of you. But it was also a thoughtful reminder that a life well lived is so very lovely.

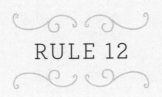

RULE 12

Practice, Practice, Practice!

When I made the decision to give my husband a year of daily intimacy for his fortieth birthday, I knew it was a bold (and borderline insane) decision. What I didn't know was that it was the first in a series of insanely bold decisions that would not necessarily alter the trajectory of my life, but would definitely transform my outlook on it.

The decision of the gift so fundamentally changed my marriage that I followed it with a crazy decision to write a book about it. The crazy decision to write the book pushed a sensitive topic to the center of a national discussion, and me with it. The supremely naive decision to try to ride the roller coaster of public dialogue and public scrutiny triggered a maelstrom of angst, doubt and personal introspection which set in motion a decision to make some changes and to ask some difficult questions about appearances, attractiveness, acceptance and effort.

And like marital intimacy, the pursuit of pretty is a personal one. My quietly introspective and unfailingly solid husband summed up our year of marital intimacy with this insightful nugget. "Intimacy every day is not a long-term sustainable model, but neither is intimacy hardly ever." The key was to land somewhere in the middle of that continuum, which is hard to determine if you're not taking notice. It's the same with getting and feeling and acting pretty. It takes time, intention and practice and it's difficult to know where you stand if you're not paying attention or paying attention only 30 percent of the time.

What I discovered is that getting pretty can be ugly, as it requires an unflinching examination of our motivations. I found I had pretty work to do—and not just on the outside—and that my attempts to define and identify my pretty code deeply informed who I was and how I chose to engage in the world.

So what does that mean for you? Honestly, I don't know. Just like I can't tell you what your marriage should look like behind closed doors, I certainly can't tell you what your pretty should look like either. Which is likely going to disappoint some. As women, we are all champing at the proverbial bit for that elusive checklist, aren't we?

Exercise daily; drink red wine; get an annual pap smear, mammogram and mole check; try a little lipo, toy with some injectables, but don't touch your lips, ever; take a daily vitamin but don't worry about fish oil; slather yourself in sunscreen and make sure your beauty providers are all on speed dial.

Trust me, you don't want a checklist from the girl who decided to find her pretty AFTER going on the national talk-show circuit. I do lots of stuff backward.

But this is what I can tell you.

Getting pretty matters for reasons that run far deeper than we might like to imagine. It extends beyond the frivolous and the silly and, for me, speaks to authenticity, kindness, graciousness and confidence. There is power in expressing my own personal philosophy not just about how I look, but about who I am (and make no mistake, the two are inextricably linked). For better or for worse, this philosophy determines my choice of friends, how I love and treat my husband, family, and friends, how I interact with others, how I spend my time and how I view my world and my tiny but nonetheless important place in it.

So if I could offer you any advice, I would encourage you to embark on your own pretty journey. Determine what's important in your personal pursuit and then get down to the hard work of practicing it and living it and owning it. It will be hard and messy and really ugly. And totally worth it.